The International Library of Sociology

THE SOCIOLOGY OF MENTAL HEALTH

In 7 Volumes

MENTAL HEALTH
AND SOCIAL POLICY
1845 - 1959

by

KATHLEEN JONES

Routledge
Taylor & Francis Group

LONDON AND NEW YORK

First published in 1960 by
Routledge and Kegan Paul Ltd

Reprinted in 1998 by
Routledge
2 Park Square, Milton Park,
Abingdon, Oxon, OX14 4RN

Simultaneously published in the USA and Canada by Routledge
711 Third Avenue, New York, NY 10017

Transferred to digital print 2013

Routledge is an imprint of the Taylor & Francis Group, an informa business

First issued in paperback 2013

British Library Cataloguing in Publication Data
A CIP catalogue record for this book
is available from the British Library

Mental Health and Social Policy 1845 - 1959

ISBN 978-0-415-17803-7 (hbk)
ISBN 978-0-415-86417-6 (pbk)

CONTENTS

CONTENTS

APPENDICES

PREFACE

THIS book was originally planned to cover a period of a hundred years from 1845, ending perhaps on the eve of the National Health Service Act; but developments which have taken place in the mental health field since it was started have been so striking, and of such lasting importance, that it seemed logical and necessary to extend it to include the Mental Health Act of 1959. The last two chapters, therefore are not 'historical' in character, but represent an interim assessment of events which are still close to the time of writing.

The author owes a debt of gratitude to Professor T. E. Chester, Professor C. Fraser Brockington and Mr. A. B. L. Rodgers of the University of Manchester, and to Professor G. R. Hargreaves of the University of Leeds; all of whom have read the manuscript in whole or in part, and have made helpful suggestions and criticisms. Especial thanks are due to Dr. Alexander Walk, of the Royal Medico-Psychological Association, for his detailed and valuable revision of the text in the final stages. (It is only fair to add that he does not wholly agree with the conclusions drawn in Chapter 1, maintaining that 'asylum doctors' in the 1845-90 period were more enlightened than the attitude of law-makers and investigators would suggest.)

Thanks are also due to Lady Adrian, who was kind enough to make available material concerning the life and work of Dame Ellen Pinsent; and to the following, for information on the subjects specified: Dr. Barbara Hammond (sources on the life of Lord Shaftesbury); Mrs. Glyn Owens (early development of occupational therapy); Mr. Kenneth Robinson, M.P. (the parliamentary debate on mental health, February 19th, 1954); Mr. W. A. J. Farndale (material on day hospitals from his own research project); and Dr. A. J. Wilcocks (the passing of the National Health Service Act).

The University of Manchester,   K. J.
May, 1960.

INTRODUCTION

IN the first half of the nineteenth century, the tide of industrial change brought new wealth and new opportunities to a few, but squalor and hardship to many. The social problems with which small rural communities had dealt casually, but on the whole effectively, became acute in the towns, where families crowded together in conditions of dirt and disease and despair; but industrialization, if it intensified social distress, also provided the means of dealing with it. The very force of distress produced a new social conscience, a desire to tackle the age-old problems of poverty and sickness and ignorance which had largely been taken for granted by the 'reasonable man' of the eighteenth century; and new, swift communications provided the means of establishing national standards where previously only local standards had been possible.

In the third and fourth decades of the century, a series of pieces of social legislation were introduced, which embodied a common ethical principle and a common administrative principle. The ethical principle was the belief that the community had a responsibility for those who could not help themselves; the administrative principle was the concept of a national framework with a central inspectorate to enforce its standards. The great Acts of Parliament of this period—the Poor Law Amendment Act, the Factory Acts, the Public Health Act of 1848—are well-known. A lesser-known Act which embodied the same principles was the Lunatics Act of 1845.

This Act marked the end of an era in reform. Behind lay a century of appalling revelations, such as those of the Select Committee on Madhouses of 1815–16, which brought home to the general public the plight of a group of helpless people. Chained, beaten and half-starved, they lived in cellars and garrets, in prisons and workhouses, out of the public eye and the public memory. A series of reformers had forced this unpalatable story into the open in the Press and in Parliament. In York, William Tuke proved at the Retreat that the insane could respond to kindness and trust, and Godfrey Higgins defied the Arch-bishop in making public the scandals of the York Asylum. In London, a group of Members of Parliament investigated Bethlem, the oldest hospital for the insane in England, and others forced their way into the private madhouses of the London area. In Gloucester, Sir George Onesiphorus Paul set in train a series of events which led to the passing of the County Asylums Act of 1808, and the first institutions specially designed for 'criminal and pauper lunatics'. A national movement for reform started with the appointment of Lord Ashley, later the 7th Earl of Shaftesbury, to the Metropolitan Commission in Lunacy in 1828.

If any one man can be said to have embodied the social conscience of the mid-nineteenth century, it is unquestionably Ashley. His work for those who laboured in the mines and the factories, for the pathetic 'climbing boys' and for the children of the Ragged Schools was in-fatigable; but no issue occupied so much of his time and energy as the care of the insane. The appointment to the Metropolitan Commission was his first public appointment, a year after he entered Parliament at the age of twenty-seven. When he died at the age of eighty-four, he was chairman of the Lunacy Commission, and much of the failing energy of his last years was devoted to this same question.

The Act of 1845 was the crown of Ashley's early work in this field. As chairman of the Lunacy Commission, he was in a position to see that the Act was operated as he wished, and also to promote the kind of improvements which cannot be secured solely by Act of Parliament. His personal vigilance, his care for the individual patient, could have a nation-wide effect.

The prospects for the treatment of the insane seemed bright. There was a new spirit of humanity in treatment, and a tentative approach to what we would now call social therapy. Asylums were generally small communities—asylums in the original sense of the word, in that they provided a refuge from the old, bad institutions of the past. There was a new concept of mental nursing which stressed the treatment of the patient as a sick individual, not a dangerous 'case'.

Yet all this promise was not fulfilled. Fifty years later, large, soulless institutions for the reception of patients in their thousands were being built—buildings which, from their very size and structure made it almost impossible to create a sense of community. Mental nurses were still 'attendants', sometimes relying more on muscular power and intimidation than on friendliness and common sense. The bogey of illegal detention was still being raised—and as safeguards for the sane were multiplied, it became increasingly difficult to secure early treatment for those who needed it. Often, it was shameful in the public estimation to receive treatment at all.

Today, the wheel has come full circle. Since the turn of the century, we have regained the social view of mental disorder. We are again beginning to think in terms of small therapeutic communities, of group work with patients, of mental nurses who are able to help the patient with his emotional and personal difficulties rather than simply caring for his physical needs. A major change in public attitudes has led in 1959 to a comprehensive Mental Health Act—a land-mark only comparable to the original Lunatics' Act of 1845.

This survey of the period between the two Acts is not exhaustive. Little is said about child guidance clinics—an important and interesting development worthy of a separate study; or about the theory and practice of psycho-analytic techniques, or the growth of psychosomatic medicine, two major factors which require a separate kind of study, written from a medical stand-point; or about the complicated legal issues relating to criminal insanity or the property of mental patients. The purpose of the survey is simply to show how succeeding generations have answered a series of fundamental questions What is mental disorder? What forms of care should the community provide? Who should be responsible for administering them? How far is it necessary to compel patients to receive treatment against their will? How can this be done without infringing the essential liberty of the subject?

As the Royal Commission on Mental Illness and Mental Deficiency pointed out in 1957, these simple questions need complex answers. We have not found all the answers yet, but the Mental Health Act of 1959 gives us a new starting-point. This book is an account of how the promise of 1845 was lost, and then recaptured in a new setting in our own generation.

PART ONE
The Triumph of Legalism

Chapter One

PUBLIC OPINION AND THE LIBERTY
OF THE SUBJECT

BEFORE 1845, there was no single code for the treatment of the insane. Subscription hospitals, such as Bethlem in London, the York Retreat, and the Manchester Lunatic Hospital, came under no control save that of their own trustees, and were run on a charitable basis. Private asylums (which were only then losing their earlier and grimmer title of private madhouses) were inspected by the Metropolitan Commissioners in Lunacy in the London area, and by panels of visiting magistrates in the provinces. County asylums, built under the permissive Act of 1808, were developing as a new form of care, and were managed by committees of magistrates appointed at Quarter Sessions; but by 1845, there were only sixteen of them, and many of the insane remained in prisons and workhouses, under the operation of the criminal code and the Poor Law respectively. In addition, there was an unknown number of 'single lunatics'—people confined in their own homes or under the care of an attendant, for whom there was no effective protection or control.[1]

The term 'insane' had by this time generally replaced 'lunatics'; but like the earlier term, it was used to cover both the mentally ill and the mentally defective, and no distinction was made between the two categories in administration or treatment.

The position in 1845

In 1842, the Metropolitan Commissioners in Lunacy were given power to inspect all types of institutions where the insane were kept,

[1] The Madhouse Act of 1828 contained provisions for the Lord Chancellor to keep a 'secret list' of such people; but these provisions were administratively unworkable.

throughout the country, for the purpose of making a report to Parliament.[1] This report led to the 1845 Lunatics Act, which gave them a similar power on a permanent basis.

The Act covered all the insane except those confined in Bethlem Hospital (which remained independent of control until 1853) and those confined privately in their own homes. A new and improved form of certification, developed from that used under the Madhouse Act, guarded against collusion between the certifying doctors in the case of a private patient. The form for a pauper patient was to be signed, as under the County Asylums Act, by a justice of the peace and the Relieving Officer of the parish, but that also required a detailed statement which protected the patient.

A system of record-keeping ensured that the Commissioners had access to information about all patients. Five sets of records were to be kept by the superintendent or proprietor of each institution, dealing with admission, diagnosis, cases of restraint or seclusion, discharge, escape, transfer or death, and reports from both official and unofficial bodies.

The purpose of the Lunacy Commission, like that of most of the inspectorates set up in this period, was two-fold. It set a minimum standard by ensuring that the provisions of the law were observed; but it also encouraged higher standards by advice and consultation, by spreading information about new methods and experiments. The Lunacy Commission and its successor, the Board of Control, have always assumed that their function is not to look coldly for flaws in administrative arrangement, but to help administrators with their problems.

To match this new administrative system, there was a wave of progress in care and treatment. By 1845, the county asylums, and the men who worked in them, were rising in public prestige. The medical profession was at this time moving towards new standards of professional competence, and among its members, the asylum doctors came to hold a special, though perhaps not a highly-honoured, place. Although there was no formal training available, there seems to have been a considerable interchange of views and experience between the members of this newly-evolving specialism. They quoted from each other's writings; they visited each other's asylums; and it was not uncommon for a doctor on first appointment to be sent to a well-known asylum to observe new methods of treatment for a few weeks before taking up his post. 'Psychology' and 'psychiatry' were new and un-

---

[1] 5 and 6 Vict., c. 87, section 7.

familiar words, but much had already been written on the medical and 'moral' management of the insane.

The old physical methods of treatment—bleeding and purging, the frequent use of intimidation to cow the patient, and leg-locks and strait-jackets to restrain him, were generally discredited. William Tuke, the pioneer in 'moral management', had proved at the York Retreat that it was possible to treat patients by social means, by trust and sympathy and simple forms of group activity. Tuke was a layman, with a deep distrust of the medical profession as he knew it at the end of the eighteenth century; and it may have been for this reason that, even when it was used by doctors, 'moral' treatment was generally held to be antithetical to physical treatment.

The logical extension of the new system was seen in 'non-restraint'—a method of treatment which involved the total abolition of all methods of restraining patients, even if they were violent. This method was first used at the Lincoln Asylum between 1839 and 1846 by Dr. Charlesworth and Dr. Gardiner Hill.

Lincoln was a comparatively small asylum, having only 130 patients; but the move was taken up at Hanwell, then the largest asylum in England, by Dr. John Conolly, perhaps the greatest asylum administrator of this period. Conolly's decision was a courageous one, for he had 1,000 patients under his care. Charlesworth and Gardiner Hill had advocated that the new policy should be introduced gradually, so that the patients might be accustomed to their new degree of freedom. Conolly covered all the stages from the frequent use of coercion to total non-restraint in a period of seven weeks. Like Gardiner Hill, he realized that non-restraint involved more than simply freeing patients. It implied a whole new concept of patient-activity, since the patients could now move about freely; and a new type of nursing, since they were no longer simply objects to be guarded.

Ways of employing the patients' energies were devised. Conolly encouraged his chaplain, the Rev. John May, to start educational classes for the patients—the first systematic use of education as a means of rehabilitating mental patients. He tried to recruit a new type of attendant, who would understand something of his patients' mental condition and behaviour. Conolly was ahead of his time in suggesting that asylum nursing should be a skilled profession, depending more on intellectual and personal gifts than on a strong nerve and powerful muscles.

Much of his work was frustrated at Hanwell, where the Visiting

Committee refused to consider schemes for a training school for nurses on the grounds of expense. The education scheme also had to be abandoned; but similar schemes were put into effect at the new Surrey Asylum in 1842. Sir Alexander Morison, the visiting physician, gave lectures to both male and female attendants on the theory and practice of asylum nursing. There was an adult school for patients, organized by the matron and the chaplain, which provided instruction in reading, writing, and Bible studies. A new departure of some importance was the foundation of a Benevolent Fund, from which grants could be made to needy patients on discharge. This is the first recorded example of an interest in mental after-care.

Possibilities in 1845

After the passing of the 1845 Act, there were three possible channels for further reform. It could develop along the social and humanitarian lines laid down at the Retreat and Hanwell and the Surrey Asylum; it could develop along purely medical lines, blurring the distinction between mental and physical disorders, sharing in the great developments which characterized general medicine in the second half of the nineteenth century; or it could proceed along legal lines, piling safeguard on safeguard to protect the sane against illegal detention, delaying certification and treatment until the person genuinely in need of care was obviously (and probably incurably) insane. In the social approach, the emphasis was on human relations; in the medical approach, it was on physical treatment; in the legal approach, it was on procedure.

The movement for further reform of the law became an affair of pressure-groups—and the pressure-groups were unequal. The legal profession had been fully established for centuries. Medicine was engaged in throwing off the shackles of a long association with barbering and charlatanism, and did not achieve full status until the passing of the Medical Registration Act of 1858, which set up a register of doctors who had passed prescribed examinations. Social work and social therapy were to remain occupations for the compassionate amateur until well into the twentieth century. It is therefore not surprising that the legal approach took precedence, to be followed after 1890 by the medical approach. It is only now, when the social sciences have developed a comparable professional status, that the social approach is coming into its own again.

The 'Liberty of the Subject'

It is ironic that the major outbreaks of public concern on the matter of the liberty of the subject came after, and not before, 1845. In the earlier part of the century, there had been many cases of illegal detention, of people who were 'put away' on doubtful evidence, and kept in secrecy and personal degradation. Patients' names were changed, they were forbidden to correspond with the outside world or to receive visitors, and the conditions under which they were imprisoned were enough to make a sane man mad. Often such patients were wealthy people, and the initiative came from grasping relatives, who were able to seize the patients' money. The madhouse-keeper had a vested interest in the continuation of the 'illness', since he was able to charge a high fee for his doubtful 'care'; it was scarcely in his interest to discharge a patient while the relatives were willing to pay for his confinement.

Ashley and his small group of parliamentary reformers had done their work only too well. They had aroused public indignation in order to press for legal control over the private madhouses. By the 1845 Act they obtained it, and the worst evils of the 'conspiracy of silence' disappeared; but public opinion was now fully aroused, and would not be quieted.

It should perhaps be stressed that public indignation was not directed at the conditions under which the genuine 'lunatic' lived, and did not arise from sympathy with mental disorder. Rather, it sprang from fear; and gradually, the phrase 'lunacy reform' came to connote the protection of the sane against conditions which were considered suitable for the insane. This was a connotation with which Shaftesbury and his associates were totally out of sympathy. The Commissioners, previously the spearhead of reform, were now forced into a defensive position, and a great deal of obloquy was heaped upon them.

A body which played a prominent role in creating this hysteria was the Alleged Lunatics' Friend Society, founded by Luke James Hansard, son of the original printer to the House of Commons. The Society was formed in 1845 '. . . for the protection of the British subject from unjust confinement on the grounds of mental derangement, and for the redress of persons so confined'.[1] There was no president. By 1851, ten Members of Parliament were vice-presidents, including Thomas Duncombe, who had strenuously opposed the passing of the 1845 Act.[2]

[1] Select Committee of 1859, p. 214.

[2] *Hansard*, July 3rd, 1845. Thomas Slingsby Duncombe was a nephew of the first Baron Feversham from whom the present Earl of Feversham (see p. 140) is directly descended.

The Society's Annual Report of 1851 complained that 'the alleged lunatic may be confined, cut off from all communication with his friends, and placed in circumstances most calculated to render him insane, for thirteen weeks or more before the quarterly visit of the magistrates or Commissioners can afford him any opportunity of appeal ...'. It admitted that the Commissioners acted 'with praiseworthy vigour' in pursuance of their duties, but quoted Ashley himself as saying that the system of inspection was 'both irregular and imperfect'. It would appear from the tenour of the Report that the Society was not on good terms with Ashley, who must have found its activities decidedly embarrassing. Its members visited asylums and investigated individual cases, taking the view that any patient who was not obviously deranged at the time of the visit should be released immediately.

The 'asylum doctors' gradually organized themselves into a rival pressure-group. In 1853, Dr. Bucknill, medical superintendent of the Devon County Asylum,[1] founded the *Asylum Journal*. A year later, this publication became the *Asylum Journal of Mental Science*, and in its sixth year, the word 'asylum' was dropped from the title. The journal was the organ of the 'Association of Medical Officers of Asylums and Hospitals for the Insane', formed in 1841. In 1865, this body changed its title to the shorter, but scarcely less cumbrous one of the Medico-Psychological Association. There was a considerable amount of discussion in the journal on the subject of terminology. In 1861, the terms 'administrative psychiatry' and 'psychological physicians' were used. The subject of study was variously described as 'medical psychology' and 'physiological psychology'. Behind this play with words was a real attempt to find verbal formulae which would describe a new professional group, and a new academic discipline.

The *Journal of Mental Science*, being the official organ of the asylum doctors, was strongly pro-medical, inclined to resent any lay intervention in their field. 'Insanity is purely a disease of the brain' wrote the editor in the second issue. 'The physician is now the responsible guardian of the lunatic, and must ever remain so.'[2]

In 1859, Dr. Bucknill complained of the activities of the Press:

'The mob of newspaper writers in the dullest season have suddenly started game ... and like a scratch pack, they have opened their sweet

---

[1] (Sir) John Charles Bucknill, (1817–97). Medical superintendent of the Devon Asylum 1844–62. Lord Chancellor's Medical Visitor, 1862–76. Editor of the *Journal of Mental Science* until 1862, when Dr. Henry Maudsley became editor.

[2] *J. Ment. Sci.*, October, 1858.

melodious voices on the poor mad-doctor . . . it is a wonderful thing, this newspaper press of ours.'

He was afraid that any legislative action resulting from this action would be 'a sop to the Cerberus of public opinion'.[1]

The Amending Acts of 1853

Three amending Acts, initiated in the House of Lords by Ashley (who had become the Earl of Shaftesbury on the death of his father in 1851) were passed in 1853. They were largely uncontroversial, and did little to allay public alarm. One related to private madhouses and subscription hospitals—now known as 'private asylums and hospitals'—and provided for a closer check on the certification of patients. The second was concerned with the provision of county asylums (now 'public asylums') and the admission of patients to them. It clarified the various means by which an asylum might be set up—by the formation of a joint authority by two counties, or by a combination of public financing and private subscription. The parish medical officer was required to visit all paupers in his area four times a year, and to notify the Guardians or the overseer of those who seemed in need of mental treatment.

The third Act was concerned with Chancery lunatics—that small group of persons who had originally been specified by the Act of Edward II, and for whom a special procedure existed. This involved the trial by jury of the case of an allegedly insane person whose relatives petitioned for a declaration of insanity to prevent him from dissipating a considerable fortune. The procedure had been simplified in 1833 and 1842 by Acts which abolished the trial by jury and created special Commissioners (known after 1845 as the Masters in Lunacy) to determine the question of sanity in these cases, and to visit lunatics and idiots so found. The cost of an inquisition was still high, however, and the Act of 1853 was designed to prevent the fortune which was at stake from being consumed by legal expenses. It made possible the holding of an inquisition by a Master in Lunacy alone in cases where the petition was unopposed.

THE SELECT COMMITTEE OF 1859

Despite the provisions of these Acts, public agitation concerning the inefficacy of the lunacy laws continued. There were rumours of ill-

[1] J. Ment. Sci., March, 1959; an open letter to S. T. Kekewich, M. P. Kekewich was chairman of the Visiting Committee at the Devon County Asylum, where Dr. Bucknill was medical superintendent.

treatment at Hanwell, complaints from released patients, a constant flow of indignant letters and articles in the national newspapers. Among those vilified was Daniel Hack Tuke (1827–95)—great-grandson of William Tuke of the Retreat, and a consultant physician of some standing. He writes :

'The author himself did not escape animadversion, and was represented in a newspaper as a brutal mad-doctor using a whip upon an unfortunate patient. The charge was the offspring of a bewildered editor who was obliged to acknowledge that he had been the victim of his own imagination.'[1]

The second Derby administration, in which Spencer Walpole was Home Secretary, appointed a Select Committee of the House of Commons in February, 1859. Both Walpole and his predecessor in office, Sir George Grey, were members of this Committee. The Committee continued to sit during the subsequent Palmerston administration. The question of reform of the lunacy laws was not a party issue.

Shaftesbury gave a clear and concise picture of the working of his Act in his evidence before this commission. He considered that the law was defective, but for a series of rather unexpected reasons. The authority of the Commissioners was too limited: they had no jurisdiction over Scotland, none over patients taken abroad—he considered foreign asylums 'wonderfully inferior to our own'—and little over Chancery lunatics. He thought that the greatest single cause of insanity was alcoholism, and that the most effective measure of prevention was the formation of temperance societies. He had a sharp exchange with Mr. Tite, a member who thought that religious preoccupations led to mental instability. Shaftesbury was a power in the Church of England. 'Am I to understand the Honourable Member to ask whether religion is a cause of madness?' he retorted on one occasion.

Shaftesbury considered that the quality of the nursing and medical staff was one of the most important factors in the development of lunacy treatment. Most urgent was the problem of recruiting male and female nurses of the right type. Wages were low—in many hospitals no more than twelve guineas a year—'the wages of a housemaid'. The hours were extremely long, and the work was exacting. There was no great shortage of female nurses, because 'the tendency of woman's nature is to nurse'; few other professions were open to women and the work suited them. Good male attendants were far more difficult to recruit. Com-

[1] D. H. Tuke, *Chapters in the History of the Insane*, p. 190.

missioner W. G. Campbell, another witness, said of male asylum at-tendants, 'They are all of too low a class. They are an uneducated class.' He considered that there was truth in the assertion that they frequently used force against their patients when they could do so undetected by authority. The development of professional standards could, he thought, best be assured by the institution of formal qualifications and a higher wage-scale.

Shaftesbury urged also the importance of medical specialization—'a school for students of lunacy'. At this time, only St. Luke's Hospital in London received medical students and gave them systematic instruction in the treatment of mental disorder, since Conolly's attempts to set up a similar school at Hanwell had failed. The consideration of this question had now been made easier by the Medical Registration Act, passed in the previous year, 1858. A professional medical council had at last been set up, with power to fix an examination standard, and to make legal recognition as a 'qualified medical practitioner' dependent on reaching this standard. The terms 'doctor', 'physician' and 'surgeon' now had a clear meaning, and the way was open for further specialization. Shaftes-bury pointed out that even a trained and qualified medical man often knew no more about lunacy than a layman, and based his judgment of a patient's condition not on his medical knowledge, but on his general experience of human behaviour.

He considered that the salary scales for asylum doctors also needed re-vision. Conolly when medical superintendent at Hanwell, received only £200 a year and a house. A fair salary would be £500 or £600 in addition to residential emoluments.

Public asylums had now been provided for almost every county in England and Wales—some by joint contracting arrangements. The larger and more populous counties, such as Lancashire and Middlesex, had built more than one.

Private asylums were decreasing in number; Bethlem had finally been brought under the supervision of the Commissioners following an inspection and inquiry ordered by the Lord Chancellor in 1853; the public asylum was now the normal channel of treatment both for fee-paying patients—for whom some beds were normally reserved—and for paupers.[1]

There were still many chronic patients in workhouses, and their treat-ment was a matter of some concern. Mr. Andrew Doyle, an inspector of the Poor Law Board, stated that of 126,000 workhouse inmates,

---

[1] There were also over 100 private licensed houses at this time.

6,947 were known to be insane.[1] Mechanical restraint was still in general use. Doyle denied any knowledge of cruelty against pauper lunatics, but with hesitation and little conviction. The attitude of the Select Committee made it clear that they believed lunatics in workhouses to be subjected to restraint, cruel treatment, poor and insufficient diet, and general neglect.

The treatment of criminal lunatics was still a subject of great difficulty, but Broadmoor was already under construction, and it was hoped that this new institution would greatly relieve the pressure on Bethlem and some public asylums.

On the question of private asylums (formerly private or licensed madhouses), Shaftesbury thought that the association of the profit motive with the care of mental patients was unfortunate. 'If patients who could pay £500 or £600 a year were so plentiful that, when one was cured, another would come, the doctor would be willing to discharge as evidence of his skill. But . . . years may go by before he gets another of the same stamp.' Since he made his living out of them, the doctor was inclined to keep his paying patients as long as possible.

The position was particularly bad in relation to single patients. Shaftesbury confessed that the Commissioners had no idea how many singly confined patients existed—'and we have spent years trying to learn it.' The Commissioners could only visit a house where they suspected that a single lunatic was detained after obtaining the authority of the Lord Chancellor. The Commissioners had no assurance that the Lord Chancellor's list was accurate or up-to-date, and they were not allowed to see it, though they might ask for specific information from it. This list did not include the names of patients confined in their own homes, where no payment was involved.

The tenour of Shaftesbury's evidence, and that of the other Comissioners and Masters in Lunacy, was in direct contrast to the evidence given by the chairman and secretary of the Alleged Lunatics' Friend Society. The chairman, Admiral Saumarez, was a member of a well-known Guernsey family, and had a distinguished naval record. He was a surgeon's son and a peer's nephew. At this time he was sixty-eight years of age, and the managing of this Society seems to have been one of his primary interests in his retirement. The secretary, Gilbert Bolden, was a solicitor.

---

[1] Section 45 of the Poor Law Amendment Act, 1834, provided that *dangerous* mental cases should not be detained in workhouses. There was no machinery to ensure that quieter cases were also sent to the asylum.

Both were at pains to placate Shaftesbury by paying tribute to the work done by the Commissioners; but they made great play of Shaftesbury's admission that the system was not yet perfect, and of Commissioner Campbell's opinion that attendants still used violence against their patients. Every safeguard against illegal confinement must be devised, even though the complex mechanism involved might sometimes delay treatment in a curable case. They complained that the Commissioners would not give them power to visit alleged lunatics and asked that any justice of the peace might be empowered to grant the right to make visits.

The Report of this Committee published some figures on the incidence of insanity. At first sight, it appeared that there was a distinct increase. The total number of patients known to the Comissioners had risen from 20,611 in 1844 to 35,982 in 1858; but the report pointed out that this higher figure was due partly to the increase in asylum accommodation, and partly to the work of the Commissioners in discovering previously un-notified cases. In addition, the population was rising rapidly, and the expectation of life had lengthened as a result of increased prosperity and medical advances in the field of public health. When all these considerations were borne in mind, the increase in numbers was a reasonable one. Shaftesbury even considered that the incidence of insanity was dropping. There were certainly no grounds for believing that it was rising.

The Committee produced, in their Report of July, 1860, a series of detailed recommendations, of which the most controversial was the proposal to introduce a magistrate's order in private cases of certification.[1] This originated in the suggestion of Gilbert Bolden, the secretary of the Alleged Lunatics' Friend Society, and was to form a point of debate and bitter recrimination for the next thirty years. Shaftesbury opposed it with all the force at his command, and was successful in preventing it from becoming law in his own life-time, though the proposal was revived after his death in 1885.[2]

In theory, the Committee thought that it was better to lessen the legal procedures of certification and to make early treatment possible. The danger that those who needed treatment would not get it in time was greater than the danger of illegal detention; but in practice most of their recommendations were for changes of procedure which would lessen this latter danger, and thereby increase the former. They considered

---

[1] Such an order was already necessary in pauper cases.
[2] And incorporated in the Acts of 1889 and 1890. See pp. 33 and 36.

that the first certificate should be valid only for three months, the case being reviewed at the end of that time; the order confining the patient should be sent to the Commissioners within twenty-four hours (the period allowed was then seven days) and the Commissioners should visit the patient 'as soon as possible'. Section 36 of Gordon's Act (the Madhouse Act 1828), which required the petitioning relative to visit the patient every six months, was to be renewed. These last recommendations were embodied in an Act of 1862, which also consolidated previous legislation.

GRANT-IN-AID OF PAUPER LUNATICS, 1874

The Committee's expressed dissatisfaction with the plight of pauper lunatics produced no immediate national result, but eventually, in 1874, an improvement in the situation was produced by the device of a grant-in-aid from the Consolidated Fund.[1] This method had already been employed in 1846 by the Peel administration to ensure the provision of parish medical officers and workhouse teachers, following the first grants-in-aid in 1833 for educational purposes. The sum now involved was 4s. per head for each pauper lunatic removed to an asylum. This gave an incentive to Boards of Guardians to get their paupers out of the workhouse and into a centre for curative treatment.

The Lunacy Commissioners, in their Annual Report for 1875, commented that this measure:

'might be beneficial in promoting the removal to asylums of patients requiring such treatment . . . it remains to be seen whether the alteration . . . will not also have the effect of causing unnecessarily the transfer to asylums of chronic cases . . . thus rendering necessary . . . a still larger outlay than heretofore in providing additional asylum accommodation. The returns for the 1st of January tend to show that such results are not unlikely to accompany the working of this new financial arrangement.'

The introduction of this grant-in-aid marked a departure from previous practice in lunacy administration. Hitherto, although the salaries of the Commissioners (paid largely out of the monies received from

---

[1] Twenty-ninth Report of Commissioners in Lunacy, 1857. See J. Watson Grice, *National and Local Finance*, p. 57. S. Webb, (*Grants in Aid*, p. 43) gives the date erroneously as 1859.

licensing) were backed by the Consolidated Fund, and county authorities were empowered to borrow from the Fund, no central responsibility had been taken for the maintenance of any section of the insane. The grant-in-aid led inevitably to a tightening of central control.

The Lunacy Commissioners' forebodings were fulfilled to some extent. Numbers of chronic patients were transferred to county asylums, which increased their custodial role and diminished their function as centres of treatment; but this process was never completed, and even today, many border-line defectives and senile dements remain in accommodation intended for the destitute or homeless.

PUBLIC OPINION AND THE 'SENSATION NOVELIST'

In 1877, the public preoccupation with the danger of illegal detention came to a head again. Among those instrumental in fostering this agitation was Charles Reade, who published his novel *Hard Cash* in 1863.

Reade later defended himself against the charge of being 'a sensation novelist' and claimed that the novel was the result of 'long, severe, systematic labour, from a multitude of volumes, journals, pamphlets, reports, blue-books, manuscript narratives, letters and living people whom I have sought out'.

This was probably true; but he set the book in the post-1845 period (the details of methods of admission and discharge of an alleged lunatic are those laid down in the 1845 Act) and neglected to add that most of his sources referred to the scandals and revelations of the early part of the century.[1]

The book tells the story of a young man, Alfred Hardie, wrongfully confined at the instance of his father, who wished to gain control of his money. He is captured by violence, beaten, intimidated and drugged, subjected to the unwelcome attentions of the matron. When at length he manages to convince a visiting magistrate of his sanity, the process of regaining his freedom involves lengthy correspondence and legal delays. This is in every respect the story recounted in 1838 by a journalist, Richard Paternoster, who was confined for six weeks, and subsequently published his experiences in a series of articles and a book entitled *The Madhouse System*. The similarities are too strong to be merely coincidental; but much of Reade's material comes from even earlier sources.

[1] Reade's biographer, Malcolm Erwin, writes that Reade 'habitually forgot to date his letters' (*Charles Reade—A Biography*, p. 145). The vagueness about dates may have been unconscious.

In one scene, Alfred tells the visiting magistrate that instruments of restraint are hidden in a locked room:

'Baker had not the key; no more had Cooper. The latter was sent for it: he returned, saying that the key was mislaid.

' "That I expected," said Alfred. "Send for the kitchen poker, sir. I'll soon unlock it."

' "Fetch the kitchen poker," said Vane.

'Cooper went for it, and came back with the key instead.'

This echoes a passage in the evidence of Godfrey Higgins, the York reformer, before the Select Committee of 1815. Higgins also came upon a locked door:

'I ordered this door to be opened . . . the keeper hesitated . . . I grew angry, and told them that I insisted on it (the key) being found; and that if they would not find it, I could find a key at the kitchen fireside, namely, the poker. Upon that, the key was immediately brought.'

At another point, Alfred is made to say:

'one or two gentlemanly madmen . . . have complained to me that the attendants wash them too much like hansom cabs; strip them naked and mop them on the flagstones.'

In the 1827 Report on the Condition of Pauper Lunatics in the Metropolis, evidence was given on the notorious 'crib-room cases of Bethnal Green' by an ex-patient, John Nettle, who described this process in very similar words. This single instance had raised a considerable public outcry a quarter of a century before Reade wrote his novel.[1]

Reade had certainly studied the available literature, and to this extent he could claim that his account was 'based on fact'. Most of his information referred to isolated cases of abuse—not normal practice—discovered and rectified many years before *Hard Cash* was written. He took the framework of the law as it was in 1863, but fitted into it incidents from sensational cases of the past.

The book was probably inspired by the Report of the Select Committee of 1859–60. It was published at a time when public feeling on these issues ran high; and it enjoyed considerable financial success.

Another novel dealing with the subject of insanity which was widely read at this time was Charlotte Brontë's *Jane Eyre*, first published in 1847. Here is the reverse of the picture—the lack of public understand-

---

[1] R. Paternoster, *The Madhouse System*, p. 55 also quotes an instance of this kind.

ing as to the real issues involved in insanity. No appeal for sympathy is made on behalf of the first Mrs. Rochester. She remains 'the monster', 'the maniac'—a grim and hated figure locked in a tower with a gin-sodden attendant. No Commissioner visits her—for, as a lunatic confined in her own home, she is outside their jurisdiction. Even those living in the same house only suspect her existence. The blanket of secrecy is complete.

Charlotte Brontë, the most 'moral' of Victorian writers, directs her sympathies elsewhere—to Jane and Mr. Rochester. It is with the greatest satisfaction, that author and reader reach the final dénouement—the fire, the death of the 'maniac' as she hurls herself from the burning building, and Rochester's freedom to marry Jane. There was some contemporary criticism of Rochester's character directed against the fact that he was a potential bigamist; but apparently not of his failure to take adequate care of his first wife.

There is no evidence in the Brontë biographies that Charlotte had ever come into close personal contact with the problem of insanity, and the character of the 'maniac' seems to be merely a figment of the imagination stimulated by the horror novels of the late eighteenth century. Mrs. Rochester is a figure from *The Castle of Otranto* or the later 'penny dreadfuls'—not a personification of an existing social problem; but when all this has been said, the fact remains that not only the author but apparently the readers also found this presentation of an insane person acceptable. Even Swinburne, writing in the 1890's, had no fault to find on this score.[1]

We may contrast with this grim picture the gentle sketch of Anne Catherick drawn by Wilkie Collins in *The Woman in White*, first published in 1869. 'Poor, dazed Anne Catherick' is mentally retarded, a little confused, but wholly an object of pity. When the hero assists 'the victim of the most horrible of all false imprisonments' to escape from an asylum by refusing to give information to the pursuing keepers, he carries the reader's sympathy with him. Later in the novel, when Laura, Lady Glyde, who physically resembles her, is locked in the asylum in her place, the author comments almost casually that 'any attempt . . . to rescue her by legal means would, even if successful, involve a delay which might be fatal to her . . . intellects, which were shaken already by the horror of the situation to which she had been consigned'. There is no sensational suggestion of ill-treatment; but the calm acceptance of the belief that asylums are places which would shake the mental balance

---

[1] A. Swinburne, *A Note on Charlotte Brontë*, 1894.

of a sane person, and from which release is almost impossible, is more telling than the vivid imaginings of Reade or Charlotte Brontë.

Fear and hatred of the insane, fear of those who cared for them: both were strong in the second half of the nineteenth century. All the uninformed public agitation centred on the border-line cases, where the issue of illegal detention could be raised. The activities of the Dillwyn Committee of 1877 are a case in point.

THE SELECT COMMITTEE OF 1877

On February 12th, 1877, a Select Committee of the House of Commons was appointed under the chairmanship of Thomas Dillwyn 'to quire into the operations of Lunacy Law *so far as regards security afforded for it against violations of personal liberty*'.[1]

Both Dillwyn and his associate, Stephen Cave, showed in their questions a remarkable lack of knowledge of any issues other than the legal ones involved.

'Do you consider,' asked Cave of Shaftesbury, 'that the facility with which patients are admitted to asylums is not too great at the present day?'

Shaftesbury's retort was, 'No, certainly not . . . we stated so in 1859, and we state it still more emphatically now.'

His patience was wearing thin under the strain of constant ill-informed attacks on his work. Now seventy-six years of age, he was nervous and depressed, uncertain of how long his failing power would enable him to carry on his public work. On March 11th, 1877, shortly before he was called to give evidence before this Select Committee, he noted in his diary, 'My hour of trial is near; cannot, I should think, be delayed beyond the coming week. Half a century, all but one week, has been devoted to this cause of the lunatics; and . . . the state now, as compared with the state then, would baffle description.' Now he undertook the laborious task of educating the Select Committee.

'It sounds very well,' said Shaftesbury, 'to say that persons acquainted with lunacy should be the only ones to sign certificates.' It was plausible to insist that a lengthy and detailed enquiry should take place before any citizen was forcibly deprived of his liberty; but by the time this step was finally taken, the symptoms would have to be so pronounced that a clear and unequivocal statement of insanity could be made. 'What fol-

[1] Italics not original.

lows from this course? Why, that the cases are very far advanced, and have got pretty nearly into the category of the incurable.'

The *Journal of Mental Science*, reporting his evidence, stated that 'His lordship spoke with a thorough mastery of every lunacy question about which he was asked'. Shaftesbury himself was pessimistic—in one of his self-doubting moods. 'Beyond the circle of my own Commissioners and the lunatics I visit,' runs an entry in his diary, 'not a soul . . . has any notion of the years of toil and care that, under God, I have bestowed on this melancholy and awful question.'

But the Select Committee was apparently won over. The report stated that 'allegations of mala fides or of serious abuse were not substantiated. Much of the evidence . . . amounted to little more than differences of opinion among medical men'.

'The Committee cannot help observing here, that the jealousy with which the treatment of lunatics is watched at the present day, and the comparatively trifling nature of the abuses alleged, present a remarkable contrast to the horrible cruelty . . . apathy . . . and indifference of half a century earlier.'

Shaftesbury's lesson in the history of reform had apparently not been in vain.

On the vexed question of a magistrate's order, the Committee did not 'attach any special importance to the order emanating from a magistrate'. Moreover, they felt that it was permissible for voluntary boarders, i.e. non-certified and possibly non-certifiable cases—to continue to be allowed in small licensed houses, provided that the Lunacy Commissioners were informed within twenty-four hours of reception.

This was the germ of the idea which would ultimately point the way out from the dilemma of early treatment versus legal safeguard. 'Nervous' cases had been admitted without formality to licensed houses since 1862, though their numbers were comparatively small; but a beginning had been made which would lead ultimately to the provisions for voluntary status under the Mental Treatment Act of 1930.

THE *Lancet* COMMISSION OF 1877

In the same year in which the Select Committee made its report, the *Lancet* sponsored a fact-finding commission on 'The Care and Cure of the Insane' under the direction of Dr. Mortimer Grenville, which was to take this idea a stage further. Dr. Grenville personally visited a number of asylums, both public and private, in London and the Home Counties, and produced a voluminous report which is notable for its sober judgment and unusually progressive views.

The general tone of the report expresses the author's belief that, after a period of unusual activity in which the worst abuses of the 'madhouse' system had been remedied, asylums were marking time, and in some cases regressing from the standards of 1845. At Hanwell, he found that Conolly's work had 'languished'.

'There was no open retrogression at Hanwell, but it is difficult to believe that there was any progress. Things went on very much in the humdrum way which might have been expected to succeed a period of energetic reform.'

At Wandsworth, (the Surrey Asylum p. 10) Dr. Grenville noted with approval the 'judicious practice' of visiting the wards unexpectedly by day and night, employed by the medical officers. He added, 'Everywhere attendants, we are convinced, maltreat, abuse and terrify patients when the backs of the medical officers are turned. Humanity is only to be secured by watching officials. . . .' At the same hospital, he was distressed to find that the old system of providing incontinent patients with straw palliasses instead of mattresses had been revived:

'Such a provision could only be advocated on the hypothesis—so mischievous in lunacy—that the bad and dirty habits of patients are to be regarded as incurable, instead of being eradicated by proper training.'

At Dartford, (the City Asylum, Stone House) he wrote acidly of the 'outside show' and the contrast with the 'spirit of parsimony' within.

'It appears strange . . . to charge a representative committee of the City of London with cheese-paring. Unfortunately, the evil is evident at every turn in this establishment.'

The staircases were 'cramped and draughty', the patients' clothing 'torn and dirty', the corridors 'meagre', the lavatories 'very defective'.

Bethlem and St. Luke's, the two great curative establishments of the metropolis, were both doing outstanding work; but both were 'singularly ill-adapted for the residence of large bodies of patients'; and though Bethlem was well endowed, St. Luke's was 'starved and crippled in its work in a fashion that reflects dishonour on the philanthropy of our great City firms and the wealthy classes of the metropolis'.

Lack of the personal touch, lack of money—these were the real evils of the system. The remedy was to be found in a radical change of attitude to the insane; and here Dr. Grenville's words are so strikingly in harmony with the recommendations of the Royal Commission on Mental Illness and Mental Deficiency of 1957 that it is difficult to believe that they were written eighty years earlier:

'. . . Patients labouring under mental derangement should be removable to a public or private asylum as to a hospital for ordinary diseases, *without certificate* . . . the power of signing certificates of lunacy should be withdrawn from . . . magistrates.'[1]

This was the enlightened medical opinion of 1877; it was to take the general public a very long time to learn from it.

Despite the work of the Lunacy Commissioners, the Report of the Select Committee, and the *Lancet* Report, there was no public support for early and humane treatment, and the constant allegations of illegal detention continued. The columns of *The Times* exhibit all the old fear and prejudice against the insane. On April 5th, 1877, a leading article commented that 'if lunacy continues to increase as at present, the insane will be in the majority, and, freeing themselves, will put the sane in asylums'. This bogey of the supposed increase of insanity, though officially denied, occurs again and again. On May 23rd, there was a letter signed 'A Lunatic's Victim' which deplored the tendency of the present laws '. . . . to protect the liberty of the lunatic at the expense of the lives, limbs and comfort of the sane'. Two days later came a complaint from an attendant:

'I have been cut down with a hatchet once, and shut up for three hours in the strong room of a private asylum with a patient suffering from delirium tremens, who stood 6 ft. 2 ins., hanging at my throat . . . and all for £25 a year.'

THE CASE OF MRS. GEORGIANA WELDON

These two public prejudices—the fear of the insane and the fear of illegal detention of the sane—reached a new height in 1884, through the much-publicized activities of Mrs. Georgiana Weldon.[2]

Mrs. Weldon was an extremely eccentric lady of considerable means

[1] Op. cit., vol. II, pp. 218–19. Dr. Grenville's italics.
[2] See *The Times* Law Reports, 1884, especially March 14th–April 2nd.

and some social position. Her husband, who held the position of Windsor Herald, deserted her in 1875, leaving her with a house and an income of £1,000 a year. She was a strong believer in psychical forces —it later transpired in legal proceedings that she believed the spirit of her deceased mother to have entered into her pet rabbit—and was associated with the editorial board of a journal called *The Spiritualist*. She had a favourite medium, Madame Nenier, under whose influence she frequently acted. She was said by a specialist in mental disorder to 'have peculiar ideas on the education of young children and the simplification of ladies' dress'. This was not in itself proof of insanity; the wealthy, eccentric Englishwoman is a common-place of nineteenth-century fact and fiction. Mrs. Weldon's behaviour was undoubtedly abnormal in that it did not conform to the conventions of the society in which she lived; but the question at issue was whether it was so strongly anti-social that she should be removed from that society.

Mr. Weldon, as the petitioning relative, requested Dr. Forbes Winslow, a specialist in mental disorder, to take Mrs. Weldon into his private asylum at Hammersmith. Dr. Winslow was an eminent man in his profession—what we would now call a forensic psychiatrist—who had given evidence in many murder cases on the issue of criminal insanity. He was a former president of the Medical Society of London, a member of the Medico-Psychological Association, and founder and editor of the *Journal of Psychological Medicine*.

The ensuing proceedings were almost farcical. Dr. Winslow and an attendant went to Mrs. Weldon's house. Mrs. Weldon bolted the door. A *dea ex machina* appeared, presumably through the back entrance, in the shape of a Mrs. Lowe, a discharged mental patient who was secretary of the Lunacy Laws Amendment Association.[1] As Dr. Winslow and his attendant forced an entry, Mrs. Weldon, disguised in the habit of a Sister of Mercy, left by another door in the company of Mrs. Lowe.

Here were all the ingredients of a popular *cause célèbre*: the society background, the wealthy and beautiful lady under threat of duress, the dramatic escape in disguise. Mrs. Weldon, who was undoubtedly an exhibitionist, then started a number of law-suits, with the support of the Lunacy Laws Amendment Association and the editor of *The Spiritualist*. She sued Dr. Forbes Winslow for alleged libel, assault, wrongful arrest, false imprisonment (in that she was under duress in her own house before she made her escape) and trespass. An interesting legal

---

[1] This appears to be the Alleged Lunatics Friend Society under a changed name. No records have been traced.

side-line arose from the fact that these events took place in 1877, five years before the passing of the Married Woman's Property Act. The house therefore legally belonged to Mr. Weldon. Mrs. Weldon was suing for trespass in a house belonging to her husband, a person who had entered with her husband's consent; and if she were successful any damages awarded to her would become the property of her husband.

Mrs. Weldon also sued her husband—for the restitution of conjugal rights; she sued a Mr. Betts, editor of *Figaro*, for alleged libel, in that he had published a statement to the effect that a pamphlet written by her 'could excite in the minds of decent people no other feeling than disgust'. She sued the editor of the *Daily Chronicle* for a similar libel. She sued the two doctors who signed the certificates. She hired the Covent Garden Opera House for a meeting on her own behalf, at which she distributed many copies of her own pamphlet, and sang from a box at the side of the stage. She subsequently disagreed with the management over the cost of hire of the hall, and sued an impresario named Rivière and the composer Gounod, who was associated with him, for breach of contract.

The multiplicity of these legal actions seems in itself *prima facie* evidence that Mrs. Weldon was not a normal person. Nevertheless, there was a strong public feeling that she was a very much wronged woman. Specialists in mental disorder disagreed in court concerning her mental condition. A Dr. Edmonds considered that she was an unconventional person, but sane; the unhappy Dr. Forbes Winslow considered that she was incoherent and deluded, decidedly in need of treatment.

There was never a clear judgement in this case. There were trials, re-trials and appeals. For months, the legal columns of *The Times* were filled with accounts of Mrs. Weldon's protests and eccentricities. In the end, she won some of her cases—in particular those against Dr. Forbes Winslow and the two certifying doctors; but the damages awarded must have been swallowed up in the costs.[1] The discussions on the principle of the liberty of the subject degenerated into squabbles on minor legal issues.

The Weldon issue brought the whole question of the amendment of the lunacy laws into the public eye in an atmosphere of heated debate and partisanship. The asylum doctors were the villains of the piece—the infringers of personal liberty. The editorial in the *Journal of Mental Science* in October, 1884 written by Daniel Hack Tuke, states, 'It is so

---

[1] *The Times* Law Report, December 1st, 1884. Judgement was given for £500 to Mrs. Weldon.

easy to talk glibly about the liberty of the subject, and so difficult to guard against the licence into which that too often degenerates'. Tuke continues with a reference to 'the crude views which are entertained upon this subject in some quarters . . . we think it right to ask that we may be generally credited with ordinary honesty and integrity'. This probably referred to Baron Huddleston's celebrated 'crossing-sweeper judgement' in which he stated after Mrs. Weldon's first trial:

'It is somewhat startling—it is positively shocking—that if a pauper, or as Mrs. Weldon put it, a crossing-sweeper should sign an order, and another crossing-sweeper should make a statement, and then that two medical men, who had never had a day's practice in their lives, should for a small sum of money grant their certificates, a person may be lodged in a private lunatic asylum, and that this order, and the statement, and these certificates are a perfect answer to any action.'[1]

The doctors were only too well aware of the difficulties of their own position, and of the weight of public sentiment which was mounting against them. Hack Tuke's editorial sounded a sombre note:

'Of one thing we are sure, and that is that troublous times are before those entrusted with the care of the insane. Already we know of several threatened proceedings by former patients. . . . Lunacy Law will be amended, or probably re-made, and the foundations will be laid at the cost of some martyrs.'[2]

[1] *Standard*, March 19th, 1884. Baron Huddleston was the last of the old Barons of the Exchequer. The title dated back to the days before professional judges. See *The Times*, Obituary, December 6th, 1890.
[2] *J. Ment. Sci.*, October, 1884.

Chapter Two

THE LUNACY ACT, 1890

FOLLOWING the Weldon cases, there developed a strong movement for a major revision of the lunacy laws; this brought together diverse groups and personalities—the Lord Chancellor and the legal profession working for the same ends as the Lunacy Laws Amendment Association and a variety of ex-patients with real or fancied grudges against the existing system. Shaftesbury's plea and Grenville's recommendations for early treatment and easier methods of admission and discharge were swept aside. The tide of public opinion was against them.

Selborne and Shaftesbury

The leader of the movement for tightening up the legal procedure was the Lord Chancellor, Lord Selborne, a man of outstanding personality and ability who, at seventy-two, had a subtle intellect unimpaired by age. His biographer credits him with 'a rare power of easy and persuasive speech, a learning and knowledge of affairs equally wide, profound and exact, the abstemiousness of an ascetic, a vigorous constitution and untiring energy'.[1] A less reverent contemporary, Lord Bowen, described Selborne as 'a pious cricket on the hearth'.[2] Shaftesbury could match him in abstemiousness and piety, but in little else.

Shaftesbury was now a very old man, in his eighties. He noted in his diary at this time 'the sensible decline of mental application and vigour'. He was afraid that 'body and mind are falling to pieces'. His diary shows an almost incredible pressure of work—constant meetings, depu-

[1] *Dictionary of National Biography.*
[2] J. B. Atlay, *The Victorian Chancellors*, vol. II, p. 420.

tations and public dinners, a voluminous correspondence on many issues, frequent interviews with both group representatives and individuals. His days were overloaded and these engagements took their toll in mental and nervous exhaustion. Between public functions, he would collapse, afraid that the next would be his last: and one comment in conversation, quoted by Hodder, comes from the heart—'I cannot bear to leave the world with all the misery in it.'[1]

These were the antagonists in the struggle ahead. The contrast could scarcely have been greater. Selborne described Shaftesbury in his memoirs[2] as 'my excellent antagonist', but the general tone of his references is one of patronage. He saw Shaftesbury as honest and well-meaning, but tiresome and politically inept. They had clashed frequently in the past over religious issues: there is a slightly acrimonious correspondence between them in The Times as early as 1842. Selborne, though not a Puseyite, was a convinced High-Churchman. Shaftesbury had broken with his cousin Pusey over the Oxford Movement and was an equally convinced Evangelical. Under the Palmerston administration Shaftesbury, as the Prime Minister's son-in-law, had been instrumental in securing the appointment of exclusively Evangelical bishops —a fact of which Selborne frequently complained in the Press and in the House of Lords.

Parliamentary Procedure 1884–9

In 1883, even before the publicity accorded to the Weldon case, Selborne had introduced a Lunacy Bill in the House of Lords. This was withdrawn owing to the lack of support at the time; but on May 5th, 1884, Lord Milltown, an Irish peer and a barrister, put forward a motion that 'in the opinion of this House, the existing state of the Lunacy Laws is unsatisfactory, and constitutes a serious danger to the liberty of the subject'. He referred in his speech to Baron Huddleston's statement in Weldon v. Winslow that 'a person could be confined in an asylum by anybody, on the statement of anybody, provided certain formalities were gone through . . . it was positively shocking that such a state of things should exist'.

It should be noted here that the Weldon case never came to the direct attention of the Lunacy Commissioners, since they would only have been officially notified of Mrs. Weldon's certification after her

---

[1] Hodder, Life of Shaftesbury, vol. III, p. 513.
[2] Memoirs Personal and Political. Roundell Palmer, 1st Earl of Selborne.

reception into Dr. Winslow's house. Since she 'escaped', this eventuality never occurred. However, Mrs. Weldon subpoenaed them in her case against Dr. Semple, one of the certifying doctors, and later commented that 'Lord Shaftesbury . . . seemed not to care much for the judge's opinions'.[1]

Milltown described the state of the lunacy laws as 'intolerable . . . a damning blot . . . (on) the Statute Book'.[2]

Shaftesbury rose to reply. He 'thought it necessary, and almost a point of duty, to explain the state of things and calm the public mind'. He deprecated Baron Huddleston's strictures, and declared that, although some revision in the law respecting private asylums was necessary, an increase in legal formality—particularly by the device of a magistrate's order—was undesirable.

Milltown's motion was carried—to Shaftesbury's great distress. A long correspondence between Shaftesbury and Selborne ensued, but there was no possibility of compromise between them. In 1885, Selborne introduced a Lunacy Amendment Bill into the Lords, and Shaftesbury thereupon tendered his resignation from the chairmanship of the Lunacy Commission.

In June, the Bill was shelved and Shaftesbury was persuaded to remain in office. The shelving of the Bill may have been due to genuine pressure of parliamentary business; to the obstruction of the Irish members —who at this time were blocking all legislation to the point where it was almost impossible to get a Bill through the Lower House; to Shaftesbury's great reputation with the general public; or to a combination of all three.

In July, Shaftesbury moved to Folkestone, and it became clear that his life would end there. He died on October 1st. Over two hundred philanthropic organizations sent deputations to the memorial service at Westminster Abbey; but the Lunacy Laws Amendment Association does not appear to have been represented.

In the session 1885–6, political conditions were unsettled, and there was no opportunity for the re-presentation of the Bill; but in August, 1886, the position was more favourable. The Salisbury administration was formed, with Lord Halsbury securely on the Woolsack. Halsbury had practised before Selborne as an advocate, and sat with him as a judge. The link between them was a strong one.

Now that Shaftesbury was gone, the way was open for the intro-

---

[1] *The Times*, July 11th, 1884. Winslow *v*. Semple.
[2] *Hansard*, May 5th, 1884.

duction of the measures he had so long opposed. On January 31st, 1887, two Bills were introduced in the House of Lords by Lord Halsbury. They represented considered legal opinion on the subject, and the Lord Chancellor paid tribute to the work done by his predecessors in office, Lord Selborne and Lord Herschell.[1] The first Bill was a consolidating measure, designed to draw existing legislation into a coherent whole. The second was the Lunacy Acts Amendment Bill, which included a number of points raised by the Dillwyn Committee, ten years before, and introduced again in an amended form the highly controversial clause requiring a magistrate's order in non-pauper cases. The Commissioners, faithful to the Shaftesbury tradition, opposed the clause; but the Lord Chancellor felt that 'no alteration of the law would be satisfactory that did not make further provision for the liberty of the subject'. He proposed a compromise, whereby a magistrate's order would not be required in every case, but the alleged lunatic could require the presence of a justice if he wished to defend his sanity.

Both Bills were passed by the Lords and sent to the Commons. The Lunacy Bill survived its third reading, but the Lunacy Acts Amendment Bill was withdrawn in August by the Solicitor-General after the first reading. No reason was given for this action, and after this, both Bills disappeared from the parliamentary scene. It was apparently not the intention of the Lord Chancellor and his supporters that one Bill should pass without the other.

In February, 1888, the Lunacy Acts Amendment Bill appeared once more in the Lords. This time, it contained the provisions of both the previous Bills. The Lord Chancellor summarized the intentions of the new Bill as follows:

1. The introduction of a judicial authority for ordering the detention of a person as a lunatic. (The previous compromise had apparently been withdrawn.)

2. The provision that all orders of detention should cease to have effect unless renewed at the stated time. This placed the onus of continued detention on the shoulders of the medical profession, rather than leaving the question of discharge to their initiative.

3. Protection to medical men and others 'against vexatious actions where they have acted in good faith'. This was a gesture to the medical profession following the widespread alarm aroused by the case of Weldon v. Winslow. This clause conciliated a powerful

[1] Lord Chancellor February–August, 1886.

pressure group—the asylum doctors—who might have wrecked the Act.

4. Restrictions on the opening of new private asylums. This was a means of winning over the Shaftesburyites. Shaftesbury had written to Lord Milltown only six months before his death to say that he had not changed by one hair's-breadth his opinions of 'the danger which beset all private asylums, and of the necessity of placing the whole care of lunacy on a public basis'.

5. Consolidating clauses.[1]

The Lord Chancellor was in fact saying to the doctors 'If you want legal protection, you must take the magistrates clause,' and to the Shaftesburyites, 'If you want to reduce the number of private asylums, you must take the magistrates clause.' He concluded with an appeal to the Lower House. The Bill 'had already received very full and careful consideration in their Lordships' House; and having been adopted at some stage in its history by each party represented in "another place", it might be expected to be received in a like spirit there'.

The Bill was introduced in the Commons by Salisbury's Home Secretary, Henry Matthews, on April 24th. Two days later, the second reading was deferred on a motion by Arthur O'Connor and Dillwyn on the grounds that it was very long, and that the House had not yet had time to digest it.

On May 8th, the Earl of Milltown asked with some irritation what had happened to the Bill; and the Lord Chancellor confessed, with equal irritation, that he did not know. By June, it appeared that the Government no longer had any serious intention of proceeding with the Bill in the face of continued opposition; and in July, it was withdrawn by common agreement.

The Lord Chancellor's determination did not slacken; and in February, 1889, the Bill was introduced for the third time. It reached the Commons in April, and a close debate followed the report of the Standing Committee in July.[2]

The clause relating to the justice's order was apparently no longer a matter of controversy. Instead, discussion centred on the proposal that all letters written by patients to certain persons in authority, including the Lunacy Commissioners and the Lord Chancellor, should be forwarded to them, and that notices should be placed prominently in every asylum informing patients that they had this right of access to

[1] *Hansard*, March 2nd, 1888.
[2] *Hansard*, July 30th, 1889.

higher authority. Dr. Farquharson, Member of Parliament for Aberdeen, who had welcomed the clauses relating to the protection of the medical profession, was very much opposed to this provision. He stated that 'hanging these notices all over lunatic asylums will tend very greatly to retard the recovery of the patients, by unsettling their minds and leading them to brood over fancied grievances'. Arthur O'Connor supported him: 'Many patients spend most of their time in writing letters to the Lord Chancellor. I know of a case in which two sisters spent every day from morning to night in writing letters to the Lord Chancellor, and another in which a person was continually writing to Satan . . .'.

The Bill was eventually passed, after some reference back to the Lords, and received the Royal Assent on August 26th.

By now, the battle was over. A Lunacy Bill to consolidate all previous enactments was introduced in the Lords in the same month, but dropped because of the pressure of parliamentary business. It was revived in the next session as the Lunacy (Consolidation) Bill. The administration was weary of the whole issue, and one can detect in the speeches of the Bill's adherents an almost pleading note, a hope that the protracted controversy over a difficult issue had been ended once and for all.

'It is simply a measure of consolidation,' placated Lord Halsbury in the Lords, 'and it is hoped that every facility will be given for its passing.'[1]

'It is a consolidation Bill only,' explained W. H. Smith, the First Lord of the Treasury, in the Commons, 'and it is to the interest of the entire community that the consolidation of statutes should be effected as speedily as possible.'[2]

The long-drawn-out controversy ended on March 27th, 1890, on a note of weary facetiousness:

'Mr. J. Morley. "I hope the First Lord of the Treasury will . . . draw attention to the fact that the Opposition have afforded great facilities for the passing of this Bill."

'Mr. W. H. Smith. "I shall certainly have great pleasure in calling . . . attention to the fact that the Opposition have given the greatest possible facilities for the passing of a Lunacy Bill." '

[1] *Hansard*, March 3rd, 1890.
[2] *Hansard*, March 20th, 1890.

THE LUNACY ACT OF 1890

The Act itself is an extremely long and intricate document, which expresses few general principles, and provides in detail for almost every known contingency. Nothing was left to chance, and very little to future development. The following summary gives only the main provisions.

Administration

(*i*) *Central:* The Lord Chancellor was still the ultimate authority. He continued to be responsible for the appointment of the Lunacy Commissioners, and to receive their reports (sections 150–62). He appointed the Chancery Visitors (sections 163–8, 183–6) and possessed direct powers of intervention, through the agency of the Lunacy Commissioners, in the affairs of single patients (sections 198–200, 206).

The Lunacy Commissioners and their secretariat continued to exercise powers of visitation and inspection over all institutions (sections 187–206) and all patients except Chancery lunatics (sections 183–6).

The Judge and Masters in Lunacy and the Chancery Visitors continued to be responsible for Chancery cases, i.e. lunatics so found by inquisition (sections 163–8, 183–6).

(*ii*) *Local:* The local authority responsible for public asylums was now the county or county borough council, as constituted under the Local Government Act of 1888 (section 240). They were compelled to build and maintain an asylum, either alone or under a joint agreement with a neighbouring authority (sections 238, 241–52). The local authority appointed the Visiting Committe of an asylum. This Committee was to be formed of not less than seven members, but there were no specifications concerning their interests or qualifications (sections 169–76).

Admission

There were four methods of admission to an asylum or a licensed house:

     (i) by reception order (sections 4–8)
     (ii) by urgency order (section 11)

(iii) by summary reception order (sections 13–22)
(iv) by inquisition (sections 12 and 90–107)

A reception order on petition could be obtained in private (i.e. non-pauper) cases if a near relative or other person stating his connection with the patient petitioned a justice of the peace,[1] adducing two medical certificates. It was necessary for the petitioner to be over twenty-one years of age, to have seen the patient within the previous fourteen days, and to undertake to visit the patient (in person or by proxy) every six months.

An urgency order applied in those private cases where there was no time for a lengthy procedure of certification. The procedure involved a relative's petition and one medical certificate only, and a magistrate's order was not necessary. The total duration of an urgency order was seven days, during which time a normal reception order on petition had to be completed, or the patient discharged.

A summary reception order was the normal method of admission for pauper patients. The initiative here rested with the Poor Law Relieving Officer or the police, who were responsible for notifying a justice of the peace. Two medical certificates were necessary in addition to the justice's order.

In the case of a patient found wandering at large, the Relieving Officer or constable could detain him and bring him before a justice (section 15), or remove him to a workhouse until proceedings could be taken (section 20). The period of detention without legal certification under this clause was not to exceed 3 days.

Admission by inquisition applied only to Chancery lunatics. There were several forms of procedure, varying in elaboration and expense. The simplest was that whereby, in an uncontested case, the Judge in Lunacy could direct the Masters in Lunacy to examine an alleged lunatic and to receive evidence on his state of mind. If they considered the patient to be of unsound mind, they would issue a certificate to this effect. A 'committee of the person' would then be appointed[2] under their

---

[1] One of a special panel appointed in each area with authority under this Act; but any justice of the peace could act in the case of a pauper patient (see 'Summary Reception Order').

[2] '*Committee.*' The accent is on the last syllable. This refers to one person, not to a group.

direction to administer the estate; and the patient could be received into an asylum, or confined singly, on an order either from the Masters or from the committee of the person. If the alleged lunatic wished to contest the issue of his sanity, he could request a trial by jury. This often meant protracted litigation, and a more costly procedure.

These methods of admission had grown out of existing legislation. The procedure for reception on petition had developed from the Madhouse Act of 1828—one of Gordon's Acts; the summary reception order, involving the Poor Law Relieving Officer or the constable, had grown out of the historic section 20 of the Vagrancy Act of 1744. The procedure for Chancery lunatics had the longest heritage of all, being derived from that *Praerogativa Regis* of Edward II which is often taken as the starting-point of lunacy legislation.

Reception orders and certificates. (*i*) *Prohibited relationships* (sections 30–3). There were detailed regulations to prevent collusion between the parties responsible for the process of certification. Prohibited relationships were: first degree relatives or relatives-in-law (i.e., father, father-in-law, brother, brother-in-law, son, son-in-law, and so on); professional or business associates (i.e. partners, assistants, employers, employees); and financially-interested parties.

These relationships were prohibited between petitioner and doctor, doctor and doctor, where two medical certificates were required; doctor and manager of the institution to which the patient was sent; petitioner and manager of the institution. It is typical of the framing of this Act that the relationships are set out at considerable length. Each case is dealt with separately, and there is no attempt to frame a general principle of non-collusion.

(*ii*) *Duration* (sections 29 and 38). The medical certificates were to be signed not more than seven days before the date of the petition, or two days in the case of an urgency order.

The duration of a reception order on petition or a summary reception order was one year. It was then renewable after periods of two years, three years, five years, and successive periods of five years, on the report of the medical officer of the asylum to the Lunacy Comissioners.

Care and Treatment

(*i*) *Reports and Visitation* (sections 39, 163–82, 187–206). A complicated system of documentation and inspection was laid down. This was an elaboration of the system evolved by Shaftesbury and his colleagues for the 1845 Act. The Lunacy Commissioners were to send two of their number—one a medical practitioner and one a barrister—to every public asylum at least once a year; to every licensed house in the metropolis four times a year, with two additional visits by a single Comissioner; to licensed houses outside the metropolitan area twice a year; to registered hospitals—i.e., subscription hospitals such as the Retreat which were not run for profit—once a year. The Commissioners were to visit without previous notice, at any hour of the day or night as they saw fit. They were to make detailed enquiries concerning the construction of the building, the classification, occupation and recreation of the patients, the physical condition and diet of pauper patients, the admission, discharge and visitation of all patients, the performance of Divine Service and its effect on the congregation, and the use or non-use of mechanical restraint. The Commissioners were to lay a report giving the number of visits made and the number of patients seen before the Lord Chancellor every six months, and were to make a detailed report of their inspection, to be laid before Parliament, once a year.

In public asylums, two members of the visiting committee (i.e., in this case the committee of management) were to make a statutory visit to the asylum every two months,[1] and to lay an annual report before the local authority of the area.

In licensed houses and registered hospitals, the justices' visitors were to inspect as follows: two, one of whom was a medical practitioner, twice a year; one, twice a year. They were to be appointed by the justices at Quarter Sessions (sections 177–81).

(ii) *Mechanical Restraint* (section 40). Restraint by instruments and appliances was only to be used for the purposes of surgical or medical treatment, or to prevent the patient from injuring himself or his fellow-patients. A medical certificate was necessary for each instance of restraint, and a report book was to be kept; a copy of the records was to be sent to the Commissioners once a quarter.

(iii) *Correspondence and Interviews* (sections 41–2). All letters written by patients to certain persons in authority, including the Lord Chancellor, a Judge in Lunacy, a Secretary of State, a Lunacy Commissioner or a Chancery Visitor, were to be forwarded unopened. The Commis-

[1] The 'rota visit'.

sioners could direct that notices explaining this clause should be placed in an asylum, and could choose the actual site of the notice, to ensure that it should be seen by all private patients. Pauper patients possessed the same right of having their letters forwarded unopened, but there was no obligation on the Commissioners to ensure that they were aware of this right. This may have been because paupers' complaints were likely to be more frivolous than those of private patients; because, in the eyes of the law, they were rather less important; because there was less need for safeguards where no property was involved; or simply because, in 1890, a high proportion of pauper patients could neither read nor write.[1]

Discharge

(i) *Absence on trial* (section 55). Any two visitors of an asylum were empowered to consent to the absence of a patient on trial for as long as they thought fit. During the period of trial, an allowance not exceeding the cost of his board in the asylum might be made to a pauper lunatic. In the case of a private patient, the written consent of the person on whose petition the original reception order was made was required.

(ii) *Boarding out* (section 57). This clause applied only to pauper lunatics, who might be boarded out with a relative or friend if the Visiting Committee and the Guardians of the Union agreed. An allowance might be made as for a patient on trial.

(iii) *Full discharge:* A private patient might be discharged on the direction of the person who signed the petition for a reception order (section 72). A pauper patient might be discharged on the direction of the authority responsible for his maintenance (section 73). In either case, the medical officer of the asylum possessed a right of veto. If he considered that the patient was 'dangerous and unfit to be at large', he could issue a barring certificate (section 74).

Two Commissioners, one legal and one medical, might discharge a patient after giving seven days' notice of their intention to do so. Any three visitors could order a discharge, or any two visitors with the advice and consent of the medical officer; or, in the case of a pauper, any two visitors, if a friend or relative was willing to be responsible for the patient (sections 75–9).

---

[1] In practice, of course, most letters written by patients were forwarded unopened.

(*iv*) *Escape:* Any patient escaping from an institution might be re-captured within fourteen days. After the expiry of that period, he could not be returned to the asylum unless fresh proceedings for certification were completed (section 85).

Miscellaneous Provisions

(*i*) *Single lunatics:* The procedure for visitation and inspection of single lunatics received for profit continued as under the Act of 1845. It will be remembered that one of the defects of that Act was the lack of provision for single patients confined in their own homes, or in charit-able institutions—the 'Mrs. Rochesters' of society. Section 206 of the 1890 Act made it possible for the Commissioners to visit such a patient, and to require periodical medical reports on the patient's mental and physical condition. The Commissioner might, if they thought fit, pass on their findings to the Lord Chancellor, who was empowered to remove the patient from custody, or to secure his transfer to an asylum.

(*ii*) '*Penalties, Misdemeanor and Proceedings*': Part XI of the Act set forth at some length the penalties for non-compliance with its terms. 'Misdemeanors' ranged from obstructing a Commissioner in the course of his duty to connivance at a patient's escape. The range of penalties for each offence was laid down in terms of fines and imprisonment.

The very length of this Act singles it out from all previous attempts at lunacy legislation, and it bears the heavy impress of the legal mind. Every safeguard which could possibly be devised against illegal con-finement is there. Dillwyn's suspicions, Mrs. Weldon's accusations, Shaftesbury's doubts, Hack Tuke's fears, Milltown's wrath, and the determination of three successive Lord Chancellors helped to shape it. The result, from the legal point of view, was very nearly perfect. From the medical and social view-point, it was to hamper the progress of the mental health movement for nearly seventy years.

PART TWO
Mental Defectives

Chapter Three

'THE PERMANENT CARE OF
THE FEEBLE-MINDED'

WHEN the Lunacy Act of 1890 came into force, it applied also to mental defectives. The Act stated (section 341):
' "Lunatic" means an idiot or person of unsound mind.'
No distinction was made between the two conditions. This was surprising in view of the fact that the movement for the recognition of mental deficiency as a separate condition was then nearly fifty years old; and a permissive Idiots Act which allowed local authorities to build special asylums for 'idiots' (the terms 'idiots', 'feeble-minded persons' and 'mental defectives' were used interchangeably during this period) had been passed in 1886. It was probably a recognition of the fact that, for many years to come, mental defectives would have to be sent to asylums for the insane, because there would be insufficient specialized accommodation for them.

The pioneer work in this field had been undertaken in France, where Dr. Itard attempted the education of a wild boy discovered by hunters in the woods. Itard was at first confident that, by creating suitable environmental conditions, it was possible to turn the boy into a normally socialized being. In 1801, he published his first pamphlet, *L'Education du Sauvage d'Aveyron*; but by 1807 he had to confess at least partial failure.

This experiment led Itard to two conclusions: that there was a condition of innate defect which could be minimized, but not eradicated, by suitable training; and that some kind of special provision for cases of this kind was necessary.

In 1828, the first institute for the education and training of the men-

43

tally defective was set up in Paris. Its work quickly gained recognition, and was followed by the foundation of similar institutions in Switzerland and Germany. From 1837, Dr. Séguin undertook the development of Itard's work in Paris, working at two large hospitals, the Paris Hospital for Incurables, and the Bicêtre. Professor J. C. Flügel states categorically that 'By the middle of the (nineteenth) century, it may be said that the principle of a special training for the mentally defective was well on the way to recognition'.[1]

Early 'Idiot Asylums' in England

Development in England was comparatively slow. A small 'School for Idiots' was started in Bath in 1846 by the Misses White, but this took only four patients. The real beginning of the work in England dates from 1847, when an 'asylum for idiots' was founded at Park House, Highgate, under the patronage of the Duke of Cambridge and the Duchess of Gloucester.

'We have laboured under the appalling conviction that idiocy is without remedy, and therefore we left it without help. It may now be pronounced,' runs the somewhat floridly written brochure, 'not as an opinion, but as a fact, a delightful fact, that THE IDIOT MAY BE EDUCATED.' The institution was supported by charitable donations, 'moderate payments' being received from those with means. 'Idiots' of both sexes and any age were received, but preference was given to those who were young and suffering from the lesser forms of defect: what we would now call 'subnormal', but probably not 'severely subnormal'. The institution moved in 1855 to Redhill in Surrey, where the new building was opened by the Prince Consort, and became known as the Earlswood Asylum.[2] By 1881, it had 561 inmates.

In 1864, a similar institution, the Starcross Asylum, opened at Exeter, and four years later, the foundation stone of the Northern Counties Asylum for Idiots and Imbeciles[3] was laid at Lancaster. The Northern Counties Asylum had the Queen as its patron, and the Archbishop of York as its president. The first medical officer came from Earlswood. It accommodated 600 patients, all male, and cost £50,000 to build. Payment for patients ranged from 50 guineas per annum to 200 guineas, though a certain number of 'children of persons in narrow

[1] J. C. Flügel, *A Hundred Years of Psychology*, 1933, p. 109.
[2] Now Earlswood Hospital.
[3] Now the Royal Albert Hospital.

circumstances' were accommodated for only twenty guineas. The first patients were admitted in 1870. The Lunacy Commissioners visited in 1871, and were pleased with what they saw—though they commented characteristically that the meat was cold, and the pipes in need of lagging.

By 1881, a return of idiots (i.e. mental defectives of any grade) in public institutions totalled 29,452. Only three per cent were receiving care and treatment in institutions specifically designed for them. The rest were scattered in workhouses, lunatic asylums and prisons. Daniel Hack Tuke, writing in 1882,[1] believed that the real total was much higher—that there were many defectives whose existence was unknown to the public authorities.

In fact, history was repeating itself. Similar factors had been present when the insane as a whole were first recognized as a separate class—the personal secrecy, the public apathy, the submerged nature of the whole problem.

Sub-Committee of the Charity Organization Society, 1877

The Charity Organization Society, founded in 1868 for the co-ordination of charitable effort of all kinds, and the suppression of mendicity, was a body of some power and prestige. One member of its original Council was Sir Charles Trevelyan a former Governor of Madras, who had two great assets: a sympathy for oppressed peoples, and a knowledge of administration both from the voluntary and the statutory viewpoint. In 1875, he placed before the Council his view that the Government should intervene in the field of provision for 'improvable idiots'—and backed his opinion with a pamphlet written by himself, and a letter from the Lunacy Commissioners expressing their agreement.

A special sub-committee of the Charity Organization Society debated the question throughout the winter of 1876–7. The members concluded that special provision for this class—it was Sir Charles who introduced the term 'feeble-minded'—was urgently necessary, since they could not be cared for adequately in lunatic asylums or workhouses. Unlike the writer of the Park House brochure, they were not over-optimistic about the results of training:

'There is a large proportion of cases which, having achieved a certain

---

[1] D. H. Tuke, *Chapters in the History of the Insane*, p. 310.

improvement, are unable to get beyond this, and are indeed liable to retrogress."

Possibly only two per cent could be trained to the point where they could be socially and financially self-supporting; but given a suitable environment, almost all could be improved to some extent. Their lives could be made less burdensome, and their usefulness increased.

One outstanding fact of this report is that the sub-committee concurred with Sir Charles Trevelyan's opinion that this was a field for State action. They recommended that, as for lunatic asylums, there should be a *per capita* grant of 4s. from the Consolidated Fund, and that the asylums should be financed out of local rates. In view of the well-known antipathy of the Charity Organization Society to State action in most fields of social work, this recommendation carried extra weight.

The report pointed out that the Lunacy Acts were already wide enough in scope to allow local authorities to build idiot asylums; but that probably little or no action would be taken unless fresh legislation was introduced, since the justices had no incentive to undertake the extra expense involved.

THE IDIOTS ACT, 1886

A deputation headed by Lord Shaftesbury—who, though he disapproved of the Society's policy in other ways,[1] had supported Trevelyan on this issue from the early stages—took the report to the Local Government Board. It was eventually accepted in principle, but the results were disappointing. The Idiots Bill was so lukewarm in tone and so conservative in character that it achieved little. It passed both the Lords and the Commons without controversy, and received the Royal Assent on June 25th, 1886—six days after Sir Charles Trevelyan's death.

The Act referred to 'an idiot or imbecile from birth or from an early age'. Local authorities were permitted—but not compelled—to erect special institutions for this class of patient, the financial arrangements being similar to those in existence for lunatic asylums.[2] A medical certificate and a statement from the parent or guardian of the patient were necessary preliminaries to admission. The Lunacy Commissioners were responsible for visitation and inspection.

---

[1] E. Hodder, *Life of Shaftesbury*, vol. III, p. 235. 'It acted, in his opinion, with too great severity, and arrogated to itself the function of being able to do everything'.

[2] See p. 18.

The Act also stated specifically that the terms 'idiot' and 'imbecile' did not include lunatics. Yet four years later, the Lunacy Act of 1890 completely overlooked this distinction, continuing to treat the terms 'idiot' and 'lunatic' as synonymous. It would appear that the Idiots Act was not a success, and that few authorities availed themselves of its powers. Indeed, Mrs. Bosanquet's *Social Work in London—A History of the Charity Organization Society*, which treats of its work in this connection at some length—does not even mention the Act.

Agitation for Government Action, 1886–1904

In the ensuing period, social issues connected with feeble-mindedness became hotly debated. Was the condition a product of heredity or environment? Could it be cured by suitable training? Could it be prevented in future generations by such means as sterilization, or segregation of feeble-minded girls of child-bearing age? Should the feeble minded be permanently segregated, or could their return to the community be envisaged after a process of socialization?

The Charity Organization Society continued to amass evidence. In collaboration with the British Association, it undertook the work of surveying the mental and physical condition of London children in elementary schools and Poor Law institutions. Evidence was also gained from the Metropolitan Association for Befriending Young Servants and the National Vigilance Society on the difficulties of feeble-minded girls and young women. General Moberley, a member of Charity Organization Society and vice-chairman of the London School Board, was instrumental in the operation of the Board's special schools for the physically and mentally defective from 1892.

Seven years later as a result of experimental special classes organized by the London County Council and other local authorities, came the Elementary Education (Defective and Epileptic Children) Act, 1899, which empowered all education authorities to set up special schools or classes for defectives of school age, to board them out near a suitable school if necessary, or to provide transport for them. The school-leaving age for defectives attending these classes or schools was raised to sixteen, in order to give them an extra period of training. There was no compulsion on local authorities to make such provision. The Act was purely permissive.

The movement, which aimed at the full implementation of the Charity Organization Society proposals, developed in 1896 into the

47

National Association for the Care of the Feeble-minded.[1] The influence of this organization was largely due to the work of two women—Miss Mary Dendy, and Mrs. Hume Pinsent.[2]

Miss Dendy was a Manchester woman, a member of the School Board and the City Education Committee. Her experience in this connection led in 1898 to the setting-up of the Lancashire and Cheshire Society for the Permanent Care of the Feeble-Minded, which raised funds by public subscription, and founded the colony at Sandlebridge, Cheshire, now known as the Mary Dendy Homes. The land for this colony—twenty acres in all—was given by the David Lewis trustees, who were also responsible for founding the near-by David Lewis Colony for epileptics.

Mary Dendy believed that life-long segregation, or, in her phrase, 'permanent care', was the only answer. Her sketch of the work of the Sandlebridge Colony[3] begins firmly, 'These notes are based on the assumption that the children to be cared for are to be detained for the whole of their lives,' and she continues, 'It was determined from the beginning that only permanent care could be really efficacious in stemming the great evil of feebleness of the mind in our country. The idea at first met with much opposition . . . happily, it is now universally regarded as the proper method of dealing with the weak in intellect.'

When fully developed, the Sandlebridge Colony consisted of six residential houses, a day school, a hospital, and a farm. It contained 170 boys and 116 girls aged between five and thirty; later two other houses, Warford Hall, which took 195 women, and Manor House, which took 200 men, were added. The children received habit training and were taught to do simple tasks. Much emphasis was laid on supervision, and on full occupation for all the patients.

Mrs. Pinsent's background was a rather different one. She served on the Birmingham Special Schools sub-committee—these classes were instituted in Birmingham in 1894—and was surprised that so few children attended the classes. Visits to several schools in the area convinced her that headmasters and headmistresses often did not understand the purpose of the special class, or the type of child for whom it was intended. She gained permission to visit all 56 Birmingham schools

---

[1] For the development of earlier local voluntary agencies, see M. Rooff, *Voluntary Societies and Social Policy*, pp. 103–4.

[2] 1886–1949. Dame Ellen Pinsent, 1937.

[3] C. P. Lapage, *Feeble-mindedness in Children of School Age*, with an appendix by Mary Dendy, 1920.

herself, and personally selected 251 children for examination. The medical superintendent of a nearby asylum, when consulted, unhesitatingly certified 172 of these. Birmingham subsequently appointed a woman doctor, Dr. Caroline O'Connor, as inspector; and within a few years, the number of children in special classes had risen from 100 to 600.

This was only the beginning. From considering Birmingham children of school age only, Mrs. Pinsent began to consider the problem in a wider setting. She induced the Birmingham Education Committee to set up an after-care committee, which traced the children after school-leaving age, and tried to help them in the difficulties of social adaptation. She secured the institution of a Girls' Night Shelter; but these measures were not enough. By 1903, she had formulated a scheme advocating a 'thorough and complete scheme of State intervention', which was published in the *Lancet*.[1]

Miss Dendy was the field-worker; she knew her children, and learned how to deal with their problems. Mrs. Pinsent was the organizer. She saw a great need, and framed a limited, clear-cut objective. Finding that nothing stood in the way of its attainment save public apathy and ignorance, she marshalled her forces like a general, and organized her campaign. She wrote pamphlets and articles, circularized members of parliament and local authorities, addressed meetings and conferences. Much of the success of the movement was due to her gifts of organization.

At this point a new factor entered the situation—the views of what became known as the 'eugenic school'. To those who worked in the field of mental deficiency, the fast-growing science of genetics brought new and alarming evidence. The old, easy optimism—the belief that almost all defectives could be cured, given time and patience—had vanished. In its place grew a profound pessimism, a conviction that mental deficiency was hereditary, insusceptible to treatment and training, and a growing danger to the whole of society. Life-long segregation, and a public policy of sterilization of the mentally unfit, were seen as the only useful principles for action.

Considerable public alarm had been caused by three factors; the growth of a systematic study of eugenics, notably through the work of Sir Francis Galton;[2] the development of intelligence-testing; and, arising out of these two, the publication of family studies which purported

[1] *Lancet*, February 21st, 1903.
[2] 1822–1911.

to show that the effect of a morbid inheritance was almost inevitably social deterioration.

Galton, who was a half-cousin to Charles Darwin, and was associated with many of his evolutionary ideas, produced his important work *Hereditary Genius* in 1869, and *Natural Inheritance* twenty years later. He applied Mendel's Law to the human race, and claimed that it held good not only for physical characteristics, but also for mental ability. Just as two black-haired parents could expect to produce black-haired children, so parents of outstanding intelligence could expect to produce intelligent children. He claimed that ability of a particular kind could be transmitted—musicians sired musicians, and statesmen begat statesmen; but if this were true, then the converse was also true. The children of criminals had criminal tendencies, and the children of the feeble-minded would almost certainly be defective.

A man of outstanding ability and wide interests, Galton was to have a far-reaching influence not only in the eugenic field, but also in the now rapidly-developing fields of psychology and sociology. His was the first systematic attempt to apply statistical concepts to biological development. The danger of his method lay in the fact that it was only possible to study half the evidence. It was incontrovertible that the children of a feeble-minded mother often appeared feeble-minded, or that the children of criminals often drifted into crime; but there was no way then known of assessing the social factors involved, of deciding how far childhood environment played a part in shaping these tendencies.

Galton founded the eugenic journal *Biometrika* in 1901. Three years later, his views were sufficiently acceptable in academic and medical circles to permit him to set up his eugenics laboratory at University College, London.[1]

Galton's early work on mental testing was taken up by an American, J. McKeen Cattell, who evolved systematic statistical tests of mental processes, particularly of reaction and the association of ideas. Cattell published his first major study in 1896,[2] and exerted a considerable influence on the development of mental testing as Professor of Psychology in the University of Pennsylvania.

In 1903, this work was taken a stage further in France, when Binet published his *Étude Experimentale*. The famous Binet-Simon tests,

[1] On Galton's death in 1911, he bequeathed £45,000 to University College, London, for the foundation of the first Chair in Eugenics. His colleague and friend, Karl Pearson, became first Galton Professor of Eugenics in the same year.

[2] Cattell, 'Address before the American Psychological Association', *Psychological Review*, vol. III, 2.

which are still widely used in a revised form, were first published two years later. These tests enabled the 'mental age' of the subject to be fixed by establishing norms for each age-level.

The mental condition of a backward child might be expressed, for example, by the statement that, when his chronological age was ten years six months, his mental age was six years and three months.

The great advantage of the Binet-Simon method was that it made it possible to introduce scientific method into a field where previously only a subjective judgement was possible. It was now possible to fix a child's 'mental age' with some exactitude, and thus to make valid comparisons. It was also possible, to a limited extent, to separate acquired knowledge from innate intelligence. The danger of the method was that, in unskilled hands, it might be used to give an appearance of scientific fact where no true judgement was possible. The Binet-Simon scale necessarily defined 'intelligence' in a fairly limited way. It was perhaps not generally understood at the time that it was not an adequate guide to the whole personality, or to an individual's response to society.

The same appearance of scientific exactitude was introduced in the family studies, which were published mainly in America, but had a wide-spread influence in England. These studies attempted to assess the influence of heredity on successive generations of large families of defective stock. One of the earliest was the study of the Juke family, published by Robert L. Dugdale in 1877.[1] This was a case which began with five mentally defective sisters, one of whom was said to be known as 'Margaret the mother of criminals'. Their descendants, at the time the study was made, numbered 540 persons, and these, together with 169 people connected with them by marriage or irregular union, made the basis of the study. Among them were 128 prostitutes, 142 habitual paupers on outdoor relief, 64 workhouse inmates, and 76 habitual criminals. A later study of the Jukes was undertaken in 1915 by Arthur H. Estabrook of the Eugenics Record Office in America, who concluded that 'over half the offspring either is mentally defective or has anti-social traits'.[2]

Another famous case was that of 'Martin Kallikak senior', published in 1912.[3] Kallikak had an illegitimate son by a presumably feeble-

---

[1] *The Jukes: A Study in Crime, Pauperism, Disease and Heredity.*

[2] *The Jukes in 1915*, p. 77.

[3] H. Goddard, *The Kallikak Family*, 1912. 'Kallikak' was a pseudonym made up of 'kalos' and 'kakos', signifying the noble and ignoble parts of the family.

minded girl. This son, Martin Kallikak junior, had, in four generations, 480 descendants, of whom 143 were feeble-minded, 36 were illegitimate, 24 were alcoholics, and 33 were sexually immoral. Kallikak senior later married a normal girl, by whom he had 496 descendants. Of these, all except three were normal, and many reached high office in the state. The three failures were merely charted as being 'somewhat degenerate'.

Even Galton would scarcely have claimed that his propositions could be demonstrated with quite this clarity. Though the Kallikak case provided fuel for the protagonists of the 'eugenic idea', the evidence, at first sight overwhelming, was in fact of a very flimsy character. The feeble-mindedness of the mistress and the intelligence of the wife were taken for granted; but there was no proof, since both had died many years before concepts of mental grading had been evolved. The feeble-mindedness of the existing descendants could indeed be proved; but there was no way of proving that it was due to the Kallikak strain rather than to any of the subsequent marriage partners. If the descendants of the irregular union were socially and mentally inferior to those of the marriage, this might well be a result of the stigma of illegitimacy and lack of social opportunity; and it was at least possible that conduct which was merely described as 'somewhat degenerate' in a well-to-do relative of a high official might lead to pauperism or criminality in less fortunate circles. The Juke case is similarly open to criticism.

The results of these three kinds of research—in genetics, in intelligence-testing, and in family studies—were largely inconclusive. While medical research had a long and distinguished history, social research was in its infancy, and its methods, particularly when employed by those unaware of the inherent limitations, were of doubtful validity. Subsequent research was to show that mental deficiency was not a clear-cut entity with a single cause, but rather a description of a condition with a multiple aetiology.

ROYAL COMMISSION ON THE CARE OF THE FEEBLE-MINDED, 1904–8

At length, in response to the growing public pressure, a Royal Commission was appointed under the chairmanship of the Earl of Radnor. Its members included W. H. Dickinson, M.P., chairman of the National Association for the Care of the Feeble-Minded; Mrs. Hume Pinsent, who, in addition to her connection with the National Association, was now chairman of the Special Schools Sub-Committee of Birmingham Education Committee; and C. S. (later Sir Charles) Loch, secretary of the Charity Organization Society. Other members included a barrister, two doctors, a Lunacy Commissioner, and the manager of an inebriate reformatory.

This group deliberated for four years, and received a quantity of evidence, much of it contradictory. Their final report steered a sane and sensible course between the Scylla of 'liberty-of-the-subject' agitation, and the Charybdis of eugenic theory.

The Commission came to the conclusion that heredity was an important factor in mental deficiency; that defectives were often highly prolific; and that other social problems, notably delinquency, alcoholism and illegitimacy, were aggravated by the fact that so many defectives were allowed complete freedom of action in the community. At the same time, they were unwilling to consider sterilization as a practicable policy, insisting that the main criterion in certification should be the protection and happiness of the defective rather than the 'purification of the race', and they stressed the possibilities of guardianship in selected cases as an alternative to permanent segregation.

Mental Deficiency and Other Social Factors

There was considerable evidence to show that mental deficiency was a key factor in crime, pauperism, illegitimacy and alcoholism. Mr. Baldwin Fleming, General Inspector to the Local Government Board, stated that every Board of Guardians was familiar with the problem of the mentally defective girl who came to the workhouse, perhaps five or six times, to bear her illegitimate children. The children were nearly always defective. He instanced the following case as a typical one:

'In C. workhouse, a girl, D.F., aged 25, had come into the workhouse to be confined. . . . She had no idea what to do with her child, which was a poor, undersized little object. . . . There was no power to retain the mother against her wish, and it was stated that she would probably leave the house as soon as the child was strong enough to go out. What would be the almost inevitable result? That in a few months . . . the mother would again be pregnant.'

On the question of delinquency, the Commission received the evidence of Dr. Kerr, school medical officer to London County Council, who said he 'would like to take the fingerprints of every Special Class child, and it would probably be found that in the succeeding ten years, very many would be found under different names in the hands of the police or in maternity hospitals'. He believed that there was a great social danger in the malleability of the average defective, who was imitative and suggestible, and could therefore easily be led into crime, chronic alcoholism or sex offences by unscrupulous acquaintances.

The medical officer at Pentonville stated that in one year, 1903–4, 389 juvenile offenders had passed through his hands, and that, on the evidence of a literacy test, he considered at least 40 per cent of them to be feeble-minded. (The literacy test was, of course, an even more blunt tool than the Binet-Simon tests, particularly when compulsory education had been in operation for so short a time.) Alcohol aggravated the problem. Witnesses before the Commission considered that 60 or 70 per cent of habitual inebriates were feeble-minded; and alcohol increased their social irresponsibility, thereby increasing the possibility of criminal or sexually immoral acts. The whole set of problems formed a vicious circle. The Commission stated strongly that 'people of this type *must not* be allowed to become habitual delinquents of the worst type, and to propagate a feeble-minded progeny which may become criminal like themselves'.

Existing Modes of Treatment

Many mental defectives came within the sphere of the Poor Law authorities, as they were unable to find or to satisfy the conditions of normal employment; but there was no authority for their compulsory detention, and nowhere to send them. In the workhouses, they were mixed with the normal inmates, to the detriment of both. There was no suitable occupation for them, and the staff had neither time nor incentive to undertake systematic training. Some received outdoor relief; but they were usually in the care of their relatives, who might also be feeble-minded.

Many were to be found in lunatic asylums; for, as we have seen, the lunacy laws made no distinction between insanity and mental deficiency, and even regarded the two terms as synonymous; but this was no solution for the young defective, nor could the lunatic asylums provide suitable training and education.

By 1907, some 9,000 children had been accommodated in special classes and special schools instituted under the Elementary Education (Defective and Epileptic Children) Act of 1899; but well over half of these were in the London area, and there was little provision in the provinces. In most rural areas, there was no provision at all. The special school mechanism was, at best, only suitable for dealing with a proportion of cases for a limited period.

Many children were dismissed as being too defective to receive education. These were often locked up all day if their parents had a sense of responsibility to the neighbourhood, or were left to run the streets and get into trouble if they had not.

The more fortunate higher-grade cases went to special classes; but the Commission was by no means satisfied that they received the right kind of education in them. There was no special training for the teachers, and concentration in most schools was on reading and writing rather than on the acquisition of social skills and aptitudes.

Among the institutions which catered exclusively for defectives, the Commissioners found idiot asylums both of the educational and the custodial type. They considered the work of the Sandlebridge Colony, and Miss Dendy's view that the majority of feeble-minded children required in a suitable environment, sustained care throughout the whole day, not merely in school hours.

Recommendations

When one considers the influences which were brought to bear on them, and the general climate of medical and social opinion at the time, the Commission's recommendations were remarkably moderate and far-sighted. They enunciated a series of general principles:

(i) The need for protection. Mental defectives needed protection from the worst elements of society, and from their own instinctual responses, because they were unfitted to 'take part in the struggle of life'.

(ii) Absence of social condemnation. 'The mental condition of these persons, and neither their poverty nor their crime, is the real ground of their claim for help from the State.'

(iii) Ascertainment. It was vitally necessary that all mental defectives should be ascertained, and brought into contact with the public services.

(iv) Administration. A central authority was necessary, to work in conjunction with powerful local bodies which would assume the responsibility for individual cases.

They therefore recommended the formation of a central Board of

Control, which would consist of medical and legal members, and at least one woman; the local authorities, county and county borough councils, should have a statutory committee for mental defectives. This committee would, in each area, take over the existing responsibility for mental defectives from the Asylums Visiting Committee and the Education Committee. It would be responsible for the ascertainment of defectives, for the provision and maintenance of residential accommodation, and for guardianship in the case of those remaining in the community.

It was suggested that the certification of mental defectives, as under the Idiots Act of 1886, should take place without the intervention of judicial authority. A medical certificate and the consent of a responsible relative were all that should be required.

Segregation was endorsed; but the suggestions concerning guardianship and supervision provided the opportunity for the development of community care in the future. The more drastic policy of sterilization was not envisaged as a practical possibility.

The Effect of the Report

Precisely because it steered a middle course, the report had a mixed reception. It did not go far enough to satisfy the eugenic school—and it went a great deal too far for the opponents of certification. There were other factors to be taken into consideration, too. The Liberal administration, under Asquith's leadership, was already engaged in its struggle with the House of Lords, and there was small hope, at that time, of getting a Bill of this nature through the Upper House. In the circumstances, there was much wisdom in the Government's decision to allow public opinion to crystallize before taking action.

There was no clear mandate from the country on social action. The Report of the Royal Commission on the Poor Laws, published in the following year, showed a strong division of feeling. There was the orthodox nineteenth-century view that poverty and social deterioration were the individual's fault, and that the intervention of the public services in his affairs should be kept to a minimum. This was the view of the majority of the Commission, whose report was drafted by C. S. Loch, then secretary of the Charity Organization Society. The minority, whose report was drafted largely by Sidney Webb, were only four in number, but they commanded an influential following in the country as a whole. They believed that the social services should ensure an optimum condition of life for all citizens, and that social failure was a failure of society to provide adequate conditions of life for the individual. 'Interfere, interfere, interfere,' urged Sidney Webb. This view was strongly supported by the growing Labour movement, particularly the Fabian wing. As far as mental deficiency was concerned, both believed that the presence of mental defectives in workhouses was wrong; but the majority wished to solve the problem by the provision of special institutions for defective paupers; the minority, by setting up a special mental deficiency authority which would have no reference to the patient's financial status.

The minority view was strongly critized by Sir Francis Galton in his Presidential Address to the Eugenics Education Society in 1909,[1] on the grounds that if all the feeble-minded were assured of reasonable conditions of life, their numbers would increase more than ever; but this probably did not represent the settled policy of the society.

The Eugenics Education Society (which was to change its name in 1926 to the Eugenics Society) was founded in 1907, largely as a result of the initiative of Mrs. A. C. Gotto, a committee member of the Moral Education League. In the same year, Galton wrote to Karl Pearson, his successor at the eugenics laboratory:

'That Eugenics Education Society promises better than I could have hoped. . . . They have got a particularly bright lady secretary who acts and works hard for the love of the thing. I have not yet ventured to join it, but as soon as I am sure that it is in safe hands, I shall do so.'[2]

By October, 1908, Galton had not only joined the Society, but had become its president. In this capacity, he urged its members to form local associations in their own areas. He was largely concerned here with what he termed 'positive' eugenics—the encouragement of parenthood among 'worthy' couples, rather than with 'negative' eugenics—the prevention of parenthood among the 'unworthy'. He defined 'worth' in the eugenic sense as being a mixture of good physique, intellectual ability, and character—inferiority in any one of these qualities outweighing superiority in the other two.[3]

Galton died in 1909, but by that time the science of eugenics was firmly established, and the Society launched on its work. By 1910, Miss Dendy and Mrs. Pinsent had become members, and there was a

---

[1] First Report of Eugenics Education Society, 1909.
[2] Quoted in K. Pearson, *Life of Galton*, vol. III, p. 339.
[3] First Report of Eugenics Education Society, 1909.

considerable degree of co-operation between the Society and the National Association for the Care of the Feeble-Minded.

The National Association's own campaign was already in operation. A joint committee in support of the Mental Deficiency Bill had been formed, headed by the Archbishops of Canterbury and York, and most of the bench of bishops, in addition to many doctors, clergy and titled people. The guiding hand was still Mrs. Pinsent's. The joint committee circularized many organizations, asking that resolutions in favour of mental deficiency legislation might be sent to the Home Secretary and the local Member of Parliament. One of its pamphlets urged immediate action:

'BECAUSE at the date of the Report of the Royal Commission, there were 270,000 mentally defective people in England and Wales, of whom 149,000 are uncertified. There is for them no recognized and generally no possible means of control, although they are totally incapable of managing themselves or their affairs.

'BECAUSE 66,000 of the mentally defective are reported by the Commissioners[1] to be at the present time urgently in need of provision. . . .

'BECAUSE in consequence of the neglect to recognize and treat their condition, the mentally defective become criminals and are sent to prison; they become drunkards and fill the reformatories; they become paupers, and pass into the workhouses.

'BECAUSE they are frequently producing children, many of whom inherit their mental defect, and nearly all of whom become the paupers, criminals and unemployables of the next generation.'

Another sheet was headed 'LIBERTY—Some examples of what is done in its name', and included brief case-histories such as the following:

'H.R. A little feeble-minded girl. Turned into the streets by her father. Found by the School Attendance Officer and placed in safe keeping. Was actually starving and filthy—verminous. Horribly disfigured by burns. Her feeble-minded brother (an adult) had put her on the fire and held her there.

'C.A. A strong boy, small; high grade feeble-minded; subject to very violent attacks of temper in which he does not know what he is doing. His father murdered his mother. So far as the law goes, C.A. is "at liberty" to leave his home at eighteen.'

In 1910, the National Association for the Care of the Feeble-Minded

---

[1] i.e., the Lunacy Commissioners.

and the Eugenics Education Society joined forces in the campaign. On double-headed stationery, their secretaries wrote to every candidate in the forthcoming General Election asking:

'Would you undertake to support measures . . . that tend to discourage parenthood on the part of the feeble-minded and other degenerate types?' Many of the answers received were equivocal (e.g. 'I will support any measure for the benefit of my constituents'); but some pledged whole-hearted support.[1] This helped to prepare the ground for the introduction of the Bill in the new Parliament.

In September, 1910, Mrs. Pinsent read a paper on 'Social Responsibility and Heredity' to a Church Congress. It is interesting to see how far she had at that time absorbed the ideas of the eugenicists; for her case-histories, complete with genealogies, were modelled largely on the American family histories, such as the Kallikaks and the Jukes. There was the case of a normal man who married a mentally defective woman. Of the ten children of the marriage, three were dead, two too young for their mentality to be assessed (they were 'physically frail and verminous'); four were at a special school; and only one was normal. But Mrs. Pinsent went further than the American theorists. She found out what the community was already trying to do for this family, how far personal failure in this case was a reflection of the community's failure to help. She came to the conclusion that the community had done all that could be expected, and more. The family was constantly being visited by no less than six officials—the sanitary inspector, the health visitor, the school attendance officer, the school nurse, the local officer of the N.S.P.C.C., and the relieving officer. And in spite of all that these people had done or were doing, the family was still neglected, dirty and verminous.

Today, with our rather more developed techniques of social casework, we might find other and subtler ways of helping such a family than the frequent but fragmentary supervision of six unco-ordinated officials; but in 1910, the issue seemed a clear one. State action had failed. The whole thing was 'a tragic waste of time and money' and permanent care of such people as the mother of this family was the only answer.

So the two societies pursued their campaign, and their policies on this issue to some extent merged. Before we turn to the battle for the Mental Deficiency Act inside Parliament, there is one more factor which should be mentioned here. This was the publication in 1908 of the first

[1] Material in the library of the Eugenics Society.

edition of Dr. A. F. Tredgold's *Mental Deficiency*—a clinical text-book which, revised in successive editions, has had an immense influence as teaching-material on the development of this field. Dr. Tredgold was then consulting physician to the National Association for the Care of the Feeble-Minded, and had acted as medical expert for the Royal Commission. His authoritative study did a great deal to crystallize ideas on the subject.

Dr. Tredgold believed that there were both 'intrinsic' (hereditary) and 'extrinsic' (environmental) factors in the causation of mental deficiency; but he added, 'It is agreed by all who have studied this question that the most frequent cause of amentia is some ancestral pathological condition—morbid heredity.' He thought that mental deficiency was a clearly distinguishable condition—'Between the lowest normal and the highest ament, a great and impassable gulf is fixed'.

Time and experience were to modify these views, and a consideration of the revisions which Tredgold made in his book in subsequent editions provides a clear picture of the medical and social advances in theory and practice which have taken place. Some of these changes will be considered later; for the moment, it is only necessary to note that the first edition, coming as it did at a time when very little had been written on this subject on a sound academic basis, formed a focal point for teaching and discussion, and had a considerable impact on the reform movement.

Chapter Four

THE MENTAL DEFICIENCY ACT, 1913

THE Report of the Royal Commission on Mental Deficiency was presented in the Lords and Commons on July 16th and 20th, 1908. It had been awaited, in the Commons at least, with some impatience, private members having twice drawn the Government's attention to the lengthy nature of the Commission's deliberations and the importance of publishing an authoritative statement at the earliest opportunity.

In 1909, the question of formulating legislation was raised on a number of occasions, but queries drew only evasive replies from the front bench. John Burns, at the Local Government Board, assured a questioner on October 20th that 'The recommendations of the Royal Commission . . . will not be lost sight of by me when any such legislation is proposed'. On November 1st, the Prime Minister, Mr. Asquith, was drawn into the twin admissions that there were 'considerable difficulties in the way of legislation' but that, at the same time, he 'hoped to make a practical effort next session in the direction of legislation'. On June 13th of the following year, when the session was drawing to its close, Mr. Winston Churchill, deputizing for the president of the Local Government Board, announced that the Government was 'fully alive to the importance of this matter'.

Members, spurred on by their constituents, brought new evidence of the need for legislation. One knew of 16 feeble-minded women in Liverpool who had, between them, produced over 100 illegitimate children, 'thereby increasing pauperism, vice and crime'. Another had been told of a feeble-minded man who, in his occasional holidays from an idiot asylum, had begotten seven feeble-minded children.

Meanwhile, outside Parliament, Mrs. Pinsent and Miss Dendy were pursuing their campaign. Their influence on local authorities, on teachers, on doctors, and on taxpayers grew month by month.

Resolutions demanding legislative action began to come in from the local authorities. In February, 1911, for instance, the Council of the City of Nottingham deplored the 'inadequacy of control of the adult feeble-minded, which ... seriously reduces the mean average of the health, the intelligence, the morality and the physique of the race' and begged the Government to place in the hands of some responsible body the 'permanent control of these unfortunates'. In all, by the end of 1912, the Home Office alone had received no less than 800 resolutions from public bodies, including resolutions from 14 county councils, 44 borough councils, 110 education committees, and 280 boards of guardians. Some of these resolutions were no doubt mutually contradictory; but public opinion was roused; and it was becoming articulate.

In March, 1912, Lord Alexander Thynne[1] stated in the Commons that 'the strides which public opinion has made on this subject in the last nine or ten months are very remarkable. Even the Right Hon. Gentleman (the Home Secretary) will agree that the subject has ripened, and is now fit for legislation'. A few months later, the Home Secretary promised legislation 'very shortly'.

During 1912, two private members introduced Bills drafted by the Eugenics Society and the National Association for the Care of the Feeble-Minded. The Feeble-Minded Control Bill, which involved the assimilation of the new central powers with the work of the Lunacy Commissioners, was short-lived. The Mental Defect Bill envisaged a separate central authority for mental deficiency, and the repeal and radical redrafting of all lunacy legislation. This Bill ran into considerable opposition at its second reading from the liberty-of-the-subect school, who spoke with alarm of the grave possibilities inherent in 'capricious detention'.[2] It never emerged from the committee stage.

The introduction of these Bills may have been caused by impatience with the Government's delay; but it is possible that the Government was trailing its coat—trying to find out unofficially what was the temper of the House. This suspicion is heightened by the fact that it would not have been possible to make a parliamentary grant for administration on a private member's Bill, so that the Bills, even if passed, could not have attained their objective.[3]

---

[1] Third son of the 4th Marquess of Bath. M.P. for Bath, 1910–18. Killed in action, 1918.
[2] *Hansard*, June 10th, 1912.
[3] J. and S. Wormald, *A Guide to the Mental Deficiency Act*, p. 4.

In May, 1912, Government action came at last. A Mental Defect Bill, Government-sponsored and supported by both parties, was introduced. It drew a strong objection from Mr. Goldstone who, in a rather muddled speech, deprecated the setting up of 'some glorified Lunacy Commission which will dub the children lunatics ... at a time when they might be brought into the fighting army of labour instead of being thrown into the scrap heaps of lunatic asylums'. The Bill was subjected to considerable comment and debate, but lapsed at the end of the session.

On March 25th, 1913, the final Mental Deficiency Bill, incorporating the recommendations of the Royal Commission, and providing for the setting up of a central Board of Control which would also take over the work of the Lunacy Commissioners, was introduced by the Rt. Hon. Reginald McKenna, then Home Secretary. It was immediately attacked by Josiah Wedgwood and Handel Booth.

Of Wedgwood, his obituary in *The Times*[1] said that 'There was a quixotic strain in him, and though he could be an admirable crusader for good causes, he was often led into wild knight errantry which bewildered his friends'. The obituary spoke also of his 'fierce individualism' and his 'not infrequent errors of judgement'.

This was a case in point. Wedgwood saw the issues involved as a clear battle between oppression and freedom, black and white. He was perhaps the last true Radical in English parliamentary history. He believed passionately in freedom at all costs, and was not disturbed by a gibe of Edwin Montague's, which he repeated against himself: 'You know, Jos., you can divide politicians into two classes—those who are statesmen, and those who are agitators. *I* am a statesman. *You* are an agitator.'[2] He saw the Mental Deficiency Bill as a measure designed to confine the free, to oppress the helpless; and characteristically, he poured all the zest and vehemence of a many-sided life into what he thought to be a battle against injustice. In retrospect, one might wish that such a champion might have had a better cause.

Here is Wedgwood's own story of what happened:

'Whenever newspaper men have to fill up a personal column and remember me, they recount how *Athanasius contra mundum* fought the Mental Deficiency Bill through two all-night sittings, sustained on chocolate. I am the champion obstructionist, who left Sir Frederick Banbury and Handel Booth pale with envy.

[1] July 28th, 1943.
[2] S. Wedgwood, *Memoirs of a Fighting Life*, 1940. p. 71.

'The Bill had some merits, but it was one whereby prostitutes could be sent to feeble-minded houses to save mankind from infection. I do not know anything about prostitutes, a class now happily extinct, but I did know that this was a clear case of expediency v. justice. In 1912, I wrecked the Bill on Grand Committee and in the House... the Government reintroduced the Bill next year. When at last it got to report stage in the House,[1] I put down nearly two hundred amendments. I did fight it from 3.45 p.m. on Wednesday till 4.00 a.m. on Thursday, and from 11.00 p.m. on Thursday till 5.00 a.m. on Friday. Few took part except myself. It is quite true that on one occasion, a Tory M.P., Hohler, went out and brought me some sticks of chocolate from the bar; it is equally true that, while someone else was speaking, I dashed out to get a drink, and the Government rushed through a few lines of the Bill... but they got their Bill, and never dared to use it!'[2]

Wedgwood's attitude during this Homeric struggle was full of inconsistencies and misconceptions. He made it clear that he disliked the principle underlying the Bill, and preferred 'to put his trust in God rather than in the Home Secretary'. He thought the Government had 'followed up the suggestions of eugenic cranks' (a hit at the Galton school), and painted a picture of children being taken away in spite of paternal protests and maternal tears to be 'locked up for life'. In reply, Reginald McKenna was patient, almost courteous, and, as always, very sure of his ground. (His biographer notes that towards the end of his life, he re-read the speeches of twenty years before, and found nothing which he wished to alter.)[3] He pointed out that this was not the intention of the Bill; that certification could only take place with the parent's consent, or where the parent had clearly failed in his duty.

Wedgwood was not to be placated. He denounced the Bill as an 'illiberal, anti-democratic measure', and continued with a sneer against 'Miss Pinsent' who had 'wonderful ability, such as only ladies seem to possess these days'[4] and who had organized a nation-wide campaign in favour of the Bill. He quoted Charles Reade's *Hard Cash*[5] as evidence of the kind of abuse which might follow the passing of the Bill, and warned the House that, if it passed into law, the Bill would 'put into prison 100,000 people who are at present at liberty'.

Handel Booth, who followed him, was scarcely more logical. He

[1] May 20th, 1913.
[2] Wedgwood, op. cit., p. 84.
[3] Stephen McKenna, *Reginald McKenna, 1863–1943*, 1948.
[4] This was the period of Suffragette agitation.
[5] See p. 19.

considered it 'a pagan Bill, anti-Christian from its first line to its last'. He asked, 'What authority have you from God or Nature to interfere in this way?' and claimed that Francis Bacon's mother was a mental defective, which was proof of the non-hereditary nature of defect.

To the question of Divine authority another member retorted with 'Lead us not into temptation. . . . The temptation of these poor creatures is beyond description.' To the statement concerning Bacon, a medical member pointed out that Bacon's mother was an extremely able woman of great culture who died at the age of eighty-two after a short period of senile decay.

These were mere debating points; but replies to the charge that the Bill was illiberal and coercive came swiftly. Miss Mary Dendy wrote to *The Times* on June 3rd, 1913, describing the case of a feeble-minded child ill-treated by its parents. 'Where is the liberty for such a child as that? It is thraldom of the most horrible description.' Members rose in the House to bring repeated evidence of feeble-minded children taken from institutions by their parents when they were old enough to earn a small wage, and miserably ill-treated afterwards. There was no doubt that the general feeling of the House was in favour of a form of certification which would protect the feeble-minded against exploitation.

There was a great deal of discussion on the definition of mental deficiency. As we have seen, the terms 'mental defective', 'idiot', 'imbecile' and 'feeble-minded' had been used in a variety of contexts, often as synonyms. Many people were not clear about the distinction between mental deficiency and insanity—even Galton wrote in 1909 that 'one person in every 118 of our population is mentally defective, being either mad, idiotic, or feeble-minded'.[1] It was therefore necessary that, if effective legislation was to be introduced for these people, some clear statement as to who they were and how they were to be distinguished should be evolved. Definitions were formulated by the Royal College of Physicians and incorporated in the Mental Defect Bill of 1912. When that Bill was in the committee stage, no less than six days were spent on this question of a definition, and twenty-seven divisions were taken. In the committee stage of the present Bill, a further three days and six divisions were expended on the question. The resultant definitions were, as the Home Secretary warned, not watertight; but they were the best that could be devised in the circumstances.

[1] Galton, *The Problem of the Feeble-Minded*, 1909. An abstract of the Report of the Royal Commission of 1904–8, with commentaries.

The appointment of the Commissioners of the new Board of Control also provoked a certain amount of opposition. The Bill provided for fifteen Commissioners, of whom twelve were to be salaried Commissioners. Four of these were to be doctors, four were to be barristers or solicitors of not less than five years' standing, and one was to be a woman. Of the three unpaid Commissioners also, one was to be a woman. McKenna proposed initially to appoint only eleven, of whom eight would be the former Lunacy Commissioners, four legal and four medical. He proposed a salary of £1,800 per annum for the chairman, and £1,200 rising to £1,500 for the others. Some members considered these figures too high, and deprecated the appointment of 'a horde of salaried officials'—this phrase being used by several in succession.

The debate continued through most of July 28th and 29th. There were lengthy and exhausting arguments, and repeated divisions in which the number of 'Noes'—the supporters of Wedgwood and Handel Booth—were gradually reduced to a mere handful. Their emotion was spent, their protest over. The final division on the third reading took place at 3.15 a.m. on the morning of July 30th. There were only three 'Noes' left. The Bill was passed, and a weary House was free to go home.

The Bill was then taken to the Lords where it received hasty consideration.[1] This was the acute period of the House of Lords controversy, and the Government was determined to force the Bill through in as short a time as possible. Lord Selborne[2] complained bitterly, 'Everyone admits, whatever his opinion may be in the second Chamber controversy, that revision is one of the functions of a Second Chamber. In the conditions under which we have to work, revision is a farce. . . . The days of this House as at present composed are nearly numbered. When the new House comes into existence, I devoutly hope that it will arrange its adjournments solely with a view to its duty of revision, and not to suit the convenience either of His Majesty's Government . . . or of the House of Commons.' But the Bill was rushed through before the end of the session. The only alternative was for it to lapse, and for the whole battle to be fought again in the next session. It completed its third reading in the Lords on August 12th, and received the Royal Assent on the 15th.

[1] Lord Haldane's opening speech on the occasion of the second reading (August 7th, 1913) is an excellent summary of the whole Bill and the Government's intention.
[2] The second Earl.

THE MENTAL DEFICIENCY ACT OF 1913

Definition (section 1)

Four grades of mental deficiency were defined—idiots, imbeciles, feeble-minded persons, and moral defectives. In each case, it was necessary for the condition to have existed 'from birth or from an early age' for the patient to come within the scope of the Act. '. . . from an early age' implied that the Act was not restricted to those suffering from congenital defect, but included cases where normal development had been arrested in childhood by illness or brain injury.

Idiots, imbeciles and the feeble-minded formed three grades of rising intelligence. Idiots formed the lowest grade. They were persons 'so deeply defective in mind as to be unable to guard against common physical dangers'. The inclusion of 'physical' in this context made it clear that higher-grade defectives could require protection from mental and moral dangers; but the idiot was as lacking in the powers of self-preservation as a baby taking his first steps.

Imbeciles were those who, while not suffering from a condition amounting to idiocy, were 'incapable of managing themselves or their affairs, or, in the case of children, of being taught to do so'.

Feeble-minded persons were defined in two ways. If adults, their condition was defined as one not amounting to 'imbecility', 'yet so pronounced that they require care, supervision and control for their own protection or the protection of others'. The criterion was thus a social one; but in the case of a child of school age, the position was quite different. Here, feeble-mindedness was defined as a condition not amounting to imbecility 'yet so pronounced that they by reason of such defectiveness appear to be permanently incapable of receiving proper benefit from the instruction in ordinary schools'. In other words, the standard was an educational and not a social one.

'Moral defectives' differed from the others in kind, not in degree. They were persons who from an early age displayed 'some permanent mental defect coupled with strong vicious or criminal propensities on which punishment had little or no effect'.

'Subject to be dealt with' (section 2)

The mere fact that a patient came within the foregoing definitions was not enough to bring him within the orbit of the public authorities.

In certain circumstances, given a sympathetic and understanding guardian and a favourable environment, a defective might be capable of something approaching normal life. It was only when he was unable to be cared for in society in the normal way that he became 'subject to be dealt with'. He might be sent to an institution or placed under statutory guardianship only under the following circumstances:

1. If he was a low-grade defective (idiot or imbecile) and the parent or guardian petitioned the local authority.
2. If he was defective in any of the four grades, and under 21, and the parent or guardian petitioned the local authority.
3. If he was defective in any grade and:
   (i) neglected, abandoned, cruelly treated, or without visible means of support;
   (ii) guilty of a criminal offence, or liable to be sent by court order to a certified industrial school;
   (iii) in prison, reformatory, industrial school, a lunatic asylum or an inebriate reformatory;
   (iv) an habitual drunkard within the meaning of the Inebriates Acts, 1879–1900.[1]
   (v) If incapable of receiving benefit from attendance at a special school; if his presence in such a school were detrimental to others; of if he attained the age of 16 years after attendance at a special school, and the Board of Education certified that further care, either in an institution or under guardianship, was required.

Certification (sections 3 and 4)

The parent or guardian of an idiot or imbecile of any age, or of a defective of any grade but under the age of twenty-one, could place the patient in an institution or under statutory guardianship. Two medical certificates were necessary, one from a practitioner specially appointed by the local authority for this work. If the patient was not an idiot or an imbecile, a judicial order was also necessary.

Where the patient was neglected, abandoned, cruelly treated, or without visible means of support, the initiative lay with the magistrate:

[1] The Habitual Drunkards Act of 1879 (42 and 43 Vict., c. 19) defined an habitual drunkard as 'a person who, not being amenable to any jurisdiction in lunacy, is notwithstanding, by reason of habitual intemperate drinking of intoxicating liquor, at times dangerous to himself or herself or to others, or incapable of managing himself or herself and his or her affairs' (section 3(b)).

an officer of the local authority was responsible for bringing the case to his notice, and acting as his agent. Two medical certificates were required. Where the patient had come within the jurisdiction of the courts, he might be dealt with under a court order; and where he was already detained in one of the institutions specified under section 2, a Home Office order was necessary.

Effect and Duration of Orders (sections 5–12)

The patient was to be conveyed to an institution within fourteen days, or, if this was impossible, to a 'place of safety' within twenty-one. A '*place of safety*' was defined by section 71 of the Act as 'any workhouse or police station, any institution, any place of detention, and any hospital, surgery, or other suitable place, the occupier of which is willing to receive temporarily persons who may be taken to places of safety under this Act'.

If the patient was capable of living a protected life in the community, and a suitable guardian was available, he might be placed under a guardianship order. Whatever the actual age of the patient, this order conferred on the guardian powers and duties analogous to those possessed by a natural parent of a child under the age of fourteen years.

The original duration of an order either for institutional care or for guardianship, was one year. It might then be renewed for five years and successive periods of five years on a medical certificate. There was one exception: where the patient was under the age of twenty-one at the time of the original certification, he was to be examined on the attainment of that age by Visitors specially appointed for each county under this Act. This enabled an independent lay judgment to be made at the time when the patient, if normal, would attain his majority.

Central Authority (sections 21–6)

A Board of Control was set up, consisting of not more than fifteen members, of whom twelve were salaried members. Four were to be legal Commissioners, and four medical. These eight Commissioners were in fact the existing Lunacy Commissioners, and under section 65 of the Act, all powers and duties of the Lunacy Commissioners were transferred to the Board. As far as mental deficiency was concerned, the Commissioners of the Board of Control were responsible for the 'supervision, protection and control' of all defectives; for the supervision of local authorities in the exercise of their powers under this Act; and for the approval and inspection of all institutions for defectives; for visitation, as follows: all institutions to be visited once a year by the Commissioners, a second visit to be made either by the Commissioners or their inspectors; and every defective under guardianship twice a year by the Commissioners or their inspectors.

The Board of Control was also to 'provide and maintain' special institutions for defectives of dangerous or violent propensities. The Commissioners had an overriding power of discharge except in the case of criminals or inebriates, for whose discharge the consent of the Home Secretary was necessary. They were to make annual reports on mental deficiency work to the Home Secretary.

Under Section 41, the Home Secretary was empowered to make regulations concerning a number of matters including the following: certification; the management of institutions; classification and treatment of patients; inspection and visitation; discharge and absence from an institution on licence; conditions of guardianship; and the study of improved methods of treating mental deficiency.

Local Authorities (sections 27–33)

The local authority unit, as for lunacy, was the county or county borough council. A special mental deficiency committee was to be set up in each area, composed largely of members of the council; but having also co-opted members with special knowledge and experience on this subject. Some of its members were to be women.

The committee was to provide for:
(i) the ascertainment in the area of all persons subject to be dealt with;
(ii) the provision and maintenance of suitable institutions;
(iii) the care, through officers appointed for the task, of mental defectives in the community, including the conveyance of patients to and from institutions; the overall care of cases under guardianship orders; and the 'supervision' (this was not closely defined) of those cases where neither institutional care nor statutory guardianship appeared to be immediately necessary.

The local education committee was given special duties with regard to defectives of school age under section 31. They were made responsible for the ascertainment of such children, and for notifying the mental deficiency committee of those who appeared incapable of benefiting from instruction in special schools or classes. These duties were later linked with the Education Acts by means of the Elementary Education (Defective and Epileptic Children) Act of 1914.[1]

Effect of the Act

The Act made possible a rapid expansion and development in provision for defectives. Local authorities set up their mental deficiency committees; many of these committees financed the voluntary mental welfare associations which had sprung up in the last few years, rather than appointing officers of their own; and the Central Association for Mental Welfare, with Miss (later Dame) Evelyn Fox as secretary, came into being to encourage the implementation of the Act and to co-ordinate the work of these local bodies.

It will be noted that, in spite of the predominantly medical and educational influences which had gone to shape it, the Act conceived of mental deficiency in an adult as primarily a social condition. It might involve a clinical condition, such as cretinism or mongolism; it might involve inability to profit from education; but the ultimate test was not physical abnormality or illiteracy, but social incapacity—an inability to guard against common dangers, a failure in self-sufficiency, a need of care and protection.

The definitions, though in some ways debatable in detail, were in principle a great achievement. It is seldom possible to come to grips with a problem until there is some measure of common agreement on terminology. The fact that it was now possible to talk about the subject with some degree of exactitude was of the greatest value in the development of both social and medical research.

One of the shortcomings of the Act from a modern view-point is the lack of a preventive element in its provisions. The patient did not become 'subject to be dealt with' until he was actually abandoned, an habitual drunkard, or already within the jurisdiction of the courts. The suspicion that he was in the care of an unfit or irresponsible guardian, that he was drinking too much, or keeping bad company, was not enough to secure his protection. This was an inevitable reflection of the agitation on the score of the liberty of the subject. The patient's right (or that of his parent or guardian) to freedom of action could not be infringed until he became a social casualty.

In spite of the strong agitation for the 'permanent segregation of the

[1] See p. 72.

feeble-minded', the Act, by its careful division of the methods of protection into statutory guardianship, institutional care, and licence from the institution, made it possible for many defectives to continue living in the community while still receiving a degree of care and control.

One more feature of the Act deserves mention here: the list of matters on which the Home Secretary was empowered to make regulations. This is an example of a type of delegated legislation which has become increasingly common in the last forty years. The Act did not attempt, like the Lunacy Act of 1890, to say the last word on every aspect of the subject. It laid down general principles, and left a great deal to be decided by administrative practice. The wisdom or unwisdom of delegated legislation may be debated on administrative and political grounds; but in dealing with this new and comparatively untried field of medical and social action, the decision to delegate ensured the maximum flexibility.

The Elementary Education (Defective and Epileptic Children) Act, 1914

While the Mental Deficiency Bill was completing its stages, another Bill, designed as its complement, had also been initiated. The president of the Board of Education, the Rt. Hon. J. A. Pease, had stated as early as June, 1913, that, of 48,000 backward children of school age, only one-third would come within the scope of the proposed mental deficiency authority. Well over 30,000 were educable, or partly educable, and for these, the special schools were the proper medium of treatment.

In March, 1913, a Bill designed to deal with these children was introduced. There was already in existence the permissive Act of 1899, which enabled local authorities to set up special schools for handicapped children, and 176 out of 318 local education authorities had taken advantage of these powers. Now the right was to become a duty. The special school would serve two purposes: it would provide manual training and character training for the backward, but not ineducable, child; and it would serve as an observation centre for doubtful cases, so that those who were incapable of receiving education might be diagnosed and passed on to the mental deficiency authority. Some dissatisfaction was expressed against this Bill. Members felt that they had already assented to an expensive procedure for the welfare of mental defectives, and this new scheme seemed to some to involve overlapping and duplication of function. Reintroduced in the session of 1914, the Bill was passed after some discussion.

Chapter Five

THE GROWTH OF COMMUNITY CARE

URING the period 1914–39, parallel movements were taking place in mental deficiency work and in the care of the mentally ill. In both cases, there was a swing away from the concept of permanent detention, and a desire to find means of integrating patients more closely with the society which had previously been concerned only to reject them; but they were distinct movements, and there was comparatively little contact between them up to 1939, though the Board of Control exercised an over-riding supervision in both spheres. Even where the Board was concerned, there was one clear difference: developments in the treatment and care of the mentally ill were largely due to the initiative of statutory organizations and salaried workers; but mental deficiency work was from the outset a partnership between statutory and voluntary bodies in which often, the initiative came from the voluntary associations. The Board of Control supervised and approved. It seldom needed to initiate.

Why did the lay public, which on the whole remained untouched by the plight of the mentally ill, rally to the cause of the mentally defective? One reason is that the mental defective was generally thought of as harmless and simple, while the mentally ill person was dangerous; though he was no longer looked on as a source of supernatural power, as in the days of witchcraft beliefs, his actions were often 'unnatural', bizarre, and held a potentiality of violence. There was perhaps a certain emotional satisfaction for the philanthropic in protecting the weak and intellectually inferior, but the emotions aroused by the thought of mental illness were so painful that the whole subject tended to be blocked. The same phenomenon occurs in other branches of social work. Most social workers know that it is comparatively easy to obtain support for work in connection with children, who are generally attractive; it is much more difficult to induce the public to care for old people, who often are not.

The Central Association for Mental Welfare

This body, known until 1923 as the Central Association for the Care of the Mentally Defective, was formed in October, 1914. Its existence arose out of a public meeting called by the National Association for the Care of the Feeble-Minded, which had achieved its object in the passing of the 1913 Mental Deficiency Act, and was now ready to dissolve in favour of a broader-based association. The chairman of the new Central Association was Mr. Leslie Scott, K.C., M.P.; and the secretary was a young woman with an Oxford degree and a wide experience of social work, Miss Evelyn Fox. At that time Miss Fox was already showing the qualities which were later to make her the architect of the mental deficiency services. The first report of the Central Association notes, 'To her public zeal, her power of organization, her knowledge of the work ... is due much of the achievement we are able to record in this report.'

The executive committee of the new association included representatives from the County Councils Association, the Association of Poor Law Unions, the Associations of Education Committees, the Prison Commissioners, the Charity Organization Society, the N.S.P.C.C., and a number of religious bodies, and had a special sub-committee of eight members of parliament. A large number of public bodies and societies, in addition to individuals, became members of the Central Association.

The first report listed twenty-eight local voluntary associations which had been formed to carry out mental deficiency work, and pointed out that since many agencies, both statutory and voluntary, were concerned with defectives, there was a great need for co-ordination. Although the Central Association sometimes dealt with individual cases, it was from the first a co-ordinating and teaching body, strong enough to achieve its purposes. There was nothing like it in the field of mental illness.

Despite the outbreak of war in 1914, the work continued. Miss Fox, to quote her friend and biographer, Marjorie Welfare, 'travelled up and down the country interviewing officials, addressing meetings, holding conferences ... sparing neither time nor trouble in her efforts to convert local authorities and social work agencies. . . . She knew how to fight, and when to fight, and she never made the mistake of going into battle unprepared'.[1] By 1918, there were forty-five local voluntary associations, many of which undertook the work of ascertainment for local authorities, and carried out casework. Local authorities often felt that a voluntary worker gained the confidence of a family more easily than did a representative of Town Hall officialdom. The Central Association did valuable work in organizing training courses for teachers and social workers, and by 1918 was already advocating the setting up of occupation centres for mental defectives. In 1919, a conference of over one hundred representatives from statutory and voluntary organizations was held in London, and future annual conferences of a similar nature were planned.

Ascertainment and Accommodation

On the appointed day under the Mental Deficiency Act (April 1st, 1914) there were 2,163 mentally defective patients receiving treatment in institutions built under the Idiots Act. By the end of that year, 796 more beds had been provided;[2] but though the energies of voluntary workers were undiminished, the work of organizing statutory committees, and of building and staffing hospitals, was seriously affected by the outbreak of war. With the many new problems brought before the local authorities by war conditions, mental deficiency became a small side-issue, and consideration was postponed in many cases until the end of the war.

There were in existence thirty-eight certified institutions, of which the largest were the five original 'hospitals for idiots': the Midland Counties Institution at Chesterfield, now known as Whittington Hall; the Western Counties Institution, Exeter, known as Starcross; the Royal Eastern Counties Institution, Colchester; the Royal Albert Institution, Lancaster; and Earlswood, in Surrey. Of the others, the Mary Dendy Homes at Sandlebridge were the best known. Small homes were run by various voluntary societies sponsored by the churches and by local welfare groups.

In addition, there were special workhouses designated under section 37 of the 1913 Mental Deficiency Act, where accommodation was set aside for groups of defectives. These accounted for 560 of the known

---

[1] Marjorie U. Welfare, *Dame Evelyn Fox*, reprinted from *Social Service*, Spring 1955.
[2] Annual Report of the Board of Control, 1914.

defectives in the country. There were also certain small homes under private ownership.[1]

It was fairly clear, however, that the number of known defectives bore no real relation to the number of those actually requiring treatment; and the Board of Control directed its energies to urging the local authorities to proceed with the business of ascertainment. Some authorities were slow to do this; for the recognition of the existence of defectives in the area meant that provision must be made for them, and both buildings and staff made heavy demands on the rates. Development was also hampered by the administrative structure of the mental deficiency services. The Mental Deficiency Committee was attached, not to the Health Department, but to the Clerk of the Council's Department, which effectively cut off the treatment of defectives from the developing health services.

By 1920, 10,129 defectives had been ascertained. This was still only a proportion of the whole, and the Board thought that the real figure was about 3·55 per thousand of the population. The Board had recently sent out a circular to all local authorities. 'Eleven authorities,' they complain in their report for 1920, 'have returned no answer at all to the circulars . . . others have sent answers from which we can only conclude that their search for defectives has been perfunctory. Others show misapprehension of the questions on the form circulated, thus rendering their return of little value. Some local authorities state that their ascertainment is "complete", when the numbers returned are so small as to make it certain that many defectives must have been overlooked.'

Other local authorities had taken their duties seriously, and had prepared schemes for the institutional treatment of defectives. The usual policy was to acquire a fairly small building—sometimes a country house, sometimes only a workhouse—and, using this as a nucleus, to add small villas as they were required and as building became possible again.

Despite the work of the Central Association in encouraging adequate provision, the development of institutional accommodation for defectives was very slow. By 1927, the total number of beds provided by local authorities was only 5,301, though the number of defectives, ascertained by that time was well over 60,000. 'It is difficult,' commented the Board of Control,

'to convince members of Councils that the expense of maintaining the

---

[1] Annual Report of the Board of Control, 1914.

feeble-minded who cannot maintain themselves must eventually be borne by the community, and that it is a choice between maintenance under improper conditions in Poor Law institutions, in prisons, by out-door relief or unemployment benefit, or maintenance in institutions where they are under continuous training and care. . . . Exposed to temptations they have no power to resist, a misery to themselves and a source of danger to their neighbours, these afflicted persons should be a first charge on any civilized community.'[1]

More beds were urgently needed; but the Board was beginning to realize that there were many cases which could not, in the immediate future, be treated by hospitalization. Consequently, they turned to considering methods of community care. So strong was the influence of what might be called the Mary Dendy theory—the permanent segregation of all the feeble-minded—that community care was at first thought of as only a rather unsatisfactory expedient. During the nineteen-thirties, parallel with the development of a similar theory in the sphere of mental illness, came the gradual realization that community care was in many cases not only cheaper and more practicable, but better for the patient.

Both statutory and voluntary supervision were possible under section 30(b) of the 1913 Mental Deficiency Act, but the Board thought that both were insufficiently stressed by the Act. By 1927, eighteen local authorities had ignored the possibilities of supervision altogether, and seven more had less than five cases on their books.

'Some authorities have told us that they have not adopted supervision, as it is practically useless. At the same time, they have not sufficient institutional accommodation even to meet their most urgent needs. Under these circumstances, it seems to us wiser to use and to improve as far as possible the method of supervision.'

They recommended that local authorities should employ specially trained officers for the work of supervision and ascertainment. They suggested that supervision should be restricted to suitable cases, i.e. to those who could make a limited response to normal society under supervision; and that attendance at occupation centres and industrial centres should be encouraged.

Occupation centres were first mentioned by the Board of Control in 1922. At that time, there were 20 in existence, all run by voluntary

<hr>

[1] Annual Report of the Board of Control, 1927.

associations, and catering in the day-time for trainable defectives who lived at home. By 1927, this number had risen to 99, and over 1,250 defectives were attending regularly. The Board of Control stated that the occupation centres aimed at 'training low grade children and adults in good habits, self-control, and obedience, and at developing to the utmost their limited capacity to lead useful lives'. Those dealing with employable defectives were more properly known as industrial centres, and aimed at simple training which would make it possible for adult defectives to take up sheltered employment. Both, said the Board, were 'essentially for defectives living in good homes, and for those who can be taught to conform to ordinary social requirements'.

The Central Association was by this time providing special training courses in mental deficiency work for social workers, for medical officers, for teachers, and for occupation centre workers. Its advisers included Lord Dawson of Penn; Dr. Tredgold, whose work in the clinical teaching of subjects connected with mental deficiency has already been mentioned; Sir Norwood East, the forensic psychiatrist and Dr. Cyril Burt, the pioneer in the study of delinquency. A quarterly journal, at first rather unhappily titled 'Studies in Mental Inefficiency' had been founded, and changed its name in 1925 to 'Mental Welfare'.

THE MENTAL DEFICIENCY ACT OF 1927

Although the 1913 Act was on the whole working well, there were some respects in which it clearly needed amendment. While local authorities were responsible for the supervision and protection of defectives, they had no statutory responsibility to occupy or train them; and now that the experiment of occupation and industrial centres had been well proved, the time had come to ensure wider provision. Again, there was a need to stress the duty of supervision; for although the 1913 Act had made provision for the supervision of defectives, many authorities were still evading this responsibility.

The third point requiring amendment was brought home by the events of 1926, when there was a serious outbreak of *encephalitis lethargica*, or sleeping sickness. Where the patient had not yet reached maturity, he became in fact indistinguishable from a mental defective—intellectually backward, and often lacking in moral restraint. Yet the 1913 Act specified that the condition must have existed 'from birth or from an early age', and was generally interpreted by doctors and magistrates to exclude cases of this nature.

A Bill to amend the Mental Deficiency Act of 1913 was introduced in the Commons in 1926; but the proposed definition of mental deficiency was very wide, and the Bill was wrecked by Col. Wedgwood, who was again wearing the 'Habeas Corpus look'. In 1927, a private member's Bill was introduced by Mr. Crompton Wood, the member for Bridgwater, supported by Sir Leslie Scott.

Crompton Wood pointed out, in moving the second reading of the Bill,[1] that *encephalitis lethargica*, meningitis and frequent epileptic fits could all result in arrested development. Yet it was impossible at that time to deal with such cases under the Mental Deficiency Act unless they were very young, or unless a medical history of the first few years of life, proving arrested development at that time, was available. Clearly there had to be some age-limit. The Bill's supporters had tried to fix the age at which an adult reached maturity, and proposed the age of eighteen. He assured 'that well-known defender of the liberty of the subject, the Right Hon. and gallant member for Newcastle-under-Lyme' (Col. Wedgwood) that this proposal would not in any way interfere with the liberty of the subject.

Wedgwood, in reply, put in a strong, but unexpectedly moderate, plea for freer conditions.

'However excellent your institution may be, however carefully you may select the matrons and managers in charge, so long as you have a lock on the door, you cannot prevent suspicion of those minor cruelties, injustices and acts of arbitrary authority which may embitter the life of the inmates of these institutions. Once you have got rid of the lock, why then, your institutions, even without so much inspection, will improve, because freedom—publicity—is the cure for any inhumanity and injustice.'

This last phrase is an excellent example of the development of an idea over more than a century. 'Publicity is the soul of justice', wrote Jeremy Bentham. Richard Paternoster used the quotation in the frontispiece to *The Madhouse System* in 1838. Charles Reade took it up in a garbled form in *Hard Cash* in 1863.[2] Now, in 1927, we find the same thought again expressed in a similar context; yet the implication is different; for Paternoster and Reade used the phrase to indicate that

[1] *Hansard*, March 18th, 1927.
[2] 'Justice is the daughter of liberty.'

those believed to be insane should be able publicly to defend their sanity. Wedgwood was pleading that those who suffered from mental handicap should not be cut off from the community.

Despite Wedgwood's intervention, the general tone of the House was strongly in favour of the Bill, and it finally received the Royal Assent in December, 1927.

The Act amended the definition of mental deficiency by substituting for the expression 'from birth or from an early age' the following:

'For the purposes of this section,"mental defectiveness" means a condition of arrested or incomplete development of mind existing before the age of eighteen years, whether arising from inherent causes or induced by disease or injury.'

Section 2 of this Act amended the previous Act by stressing provision for the supervision of defectives. Section 7 added to the local authority's duty of supervision the duties of training and occupation.

The changes which the 1927 Act introduced altered the previous Act by only a few words, but the effect was to embody in the law a new idea: a widening of the definition of mental deficiency, but also a loosening of the statutory restraints. The emphasis was no longer on segregation at all costs. The system had become more flexible, and allowed for a variety of provision suited to the needs of the individual defective. He might go to an institution, or he might remain in the community; but in deciding his future, his own well-being and happiness would be the primary consideration.

REPORT OF THE WOOD COMMITTEE, 1929

There was one other problem inherent in the administration of the mental deficiency services which could not be settled by Act of Parliament. This was the question of the division of powers in dealing with defective children. Some were cared for by Mental Deficiency Committees, some by Education Committees; and often there was confusion between the two. The Board of Control urged co-operation, and suggested that such children should receive a uniform kind of care and education.

As a result, a joint committee of the Board of Education and the Board of Control was set up in June, 1924 on the initiative of Sir George Newman, then chief medical officer of the Board of Education. The chairman, A. H. Wood, was a member of Newman's own department. Other members, in addition to those representing their departments, including Professor Cyril Burt and Dr. A. F. Tredgold; Dr. Douglas Turner, a foundation member of the council of the Central Association for Mental Welfare, and medical superintendent of the Royal Eastern Counties Institution at Colchester; Miss Evelyn Fox; and Mrs. Hume Pinsent, now a Commissioner of the Board of Control.

The Committee's primary task was to answer two questions: 'How many defectives are there?' and 'What is the best way of dealing with mental defectives?' At first their terms of reference applied only to children, but early in 1925 they were extended to cover adult defectives also.

The Existing Services

The Committee began its report with a survey of legislation: the Idiots Act of 1886, and its supersession by the Mental Deficiency Act of 1913; the Elementary Education (Defective and Epileptic Children) Act of 1899, which had empowered local authorities to set up special schools and classes, and the Act of the same title, which, in 1914, transformed this power into a duty incumbent upon all authorities.

To this basic legislation had been added the Education Act of 1921. Sections 53–5 and 58 of this Act referred to defective children, and laid the following duties on the education authority:

The local education authority was to ascertain all defective children in the area, and had the right to enforce attendance at special schools and classes; though it was laid down as a general principle that the wishes of the parents should be consulted where possible.

These powers referred to all children between the ages of seven and sixteen, and meant that all the machinery of the educational system— the school medical service, the attendance officers, and so on—could be used to ascertain and deal with defectives.

The education authority was responsible for dividing the 'educable' from the 'ineducable' and for notifying the latter to the mental deficiency authority. Where there were no facilities for special education, or where a child was vicious or out of control, an 'educable' child might also be notified.

This was the outline of the scheme: the education authority provided for educable defectives between seven and sixteen, and the mental deficiency authority took care of the rest, by means of institutional care, guardianship, supervision, and in the last two cases, possibly by means of an occupation centre. On paper, it was an admirably simple scheme; but in fact, there were so many anomalies that the scheme was proving unworkable.

Anomalies in the Existing Services

The scheme might have worked reasonably well if only the mental deficiency authority had been attached to the health department, not the Clerk of the Council's department. This would have made possible a link with the School Medical Service, and thus brought the care of ineducable defectives into close administrative contact with the care of educable defectives. As it was, they were operating separately, and in fact three other types of authority were involved as well. These were the Poor Law authorities, the Lunacy authorities, and the Home Office.

Section 30 of the Mental Deficiency Act of 1913 stated, 'Nothing in this Act shall affect the powers and duties of the Poor Law authorities under the Acts relating to the relief of the poor, with respect to any defectives who may be dealt with under those Acts'. This meant that the Poor Law Guardians had no duty to report mental defectives in their care to the mental deficiency authority; and that mental defectives dealt with under the Poor Law had none of the protection envisaged by the Mental Deficiency Act. They could not be sent out on licence, transferred to guardianship, or placed under voluntary supervision. The mental deficiency authority had no power to intervene until after they were discharged from the Poor Law institution; and, since they were not certified, they might be discharged by the Guardians or withdrawn by relatives without the knowledge of the mental deficiency authority.

Local education authorities had no right of entry into Poor Law institutions, and though the Board of Control had such a right, and would use it when requested, this was not an adequate substitute for regular visitation on a local level. It was generally acknowledged that, with a very few exceptions, the Guardians made no attempt at providing suitable training and educational programmes for defective inmates.

As far as the lunacy authorities were concerned, the position was almost as complicated. Although it was possible for mental defectives to be transferred from mental hospitals to mental deficiency institutions, the acute lack of beds in the latter made this impracticable in many cases.

Mental hospitals were in the difficult position of having many patients for whom they could do nothing (since the framework and staffing of a mental hospital was not suitable for the training of defectives) while at the same time they wished to admit other patients for whom they had no beds.

The Home Office also had special powers in relation to mental defectives, since it was responsible for juvenile offenders. There was no compulsion on Home Office schools to notify the mental deficiency authority when a defective child was discharged; and the powers of the Home Office ceased when the child was eighteen or nineteen—an age at which it was sometimes exceedingly difficult to prove that a child was 'subject to be dealt with' though there might be good reason for thinking that care was urgently necessary. The mental deficiency authority had to wait, powerless, until one of the social disasters specified under the 1913 Mental Deficiency Act took place. Then, and only then, could they act.

It was thus clear that the mental deficiency authorities and the education authorities between them were dealing with only a percentage of the actual cases; and that the rest were scattered among authorities who had no real responsibility for their care. In fact, many defective children were receiving treatment not according to their condition, but according to the actual circumstances of social breakdown, which were largely irrelevant to the question of care.

The Mentally Defective Child

In fact, even where the right authorities were able to deal with the child, the system was not working well. It depended primarily on the perception and understanding of two people, the class teacher and the school doctor. There were many class teachers who had no idea what the factors in mental deficiency were, and were quite unable to distinguish between a handicapped child and one emotionally disturbed, wilfully refusing to learn. School doctors were primarily looking for physical disorders. Because of the large burden of work involved in regular medical inspections, their work was often hurried. Some thought in any case that it was useless to certify a child when there was no adequate provision in the area. (This, of course, was a vicious circle; for until the number of certified children was sufficiently high to warrant action by the mental deficiency committee, there would be no provision.) Both teacher and doctor often thought, not without reason, that there was a social stigma in certification, and avoided it wherever possible.

The position in 1929 was that 33,000 children between the ages of seven and sixteen were ascertained. This represented 6·0 per thousand of the school population. Sir George Newman had stated, shortly before appointing the Wood Committee, that he was convinced that the actual figure was in the region of 7·5 per thousand. In a special investigation sponsored by the Wood Committee, Dr. E. O. Lewis was seconded from the Board of Control to carry out an investigation. He stated that a conservative estimate would be 8·0 per thousand of the school population.

There were probably 18,000 defectives still unascertained in the schools alone; and for those who had been ascertained, there were not enough special schools. Of the 33,000 children known to be defective, 14,850 attended day special schools, and 1,900 were in residental accommodation. The rest were still in the general educational framework—profiting little, and handicapping overworked teachers in the attempt to do their real task of dealing with the educable.

The Adult Defective

Many adult defectives were being dealt with, not by the mental deficiency authority, but by authorities whose main task was to deal with poverty, insanity, or delinquency. These were thought to account for about half the adult mental defectives ascertained at that time. Dr. Lewis, in his survey, discovered that the actual position was much worse. In the six 'representative areas' he investigated, only 10 per cent of the defectives were in mental deficiency institutions. 25 per cent were in mental hospitals; 39 per cent were in Poor Law institutions. All the cases dealt with by the mental deficiency authority—by institutional treatment, by licence, guardianship, voluntary or statutory supervision—amounted to only 40,000 out of a total of 175,000.

While the Board of Control and the Central Association for Mental Welfare were priding themselves on immensely improved services, these services were touching only a fraction of the total number needing help and treatment.

The Wood Committee thought that these were problems that could be solved by administrative means and under existing legislation. They recommended that all mental defectives in receipt of out-door relief should be transferred to the care of the mental deficiency authority; that certain Poor Law institutions should be used for the grouping together of defectives, and that these should then be transferred also; and that supervision, guardianship and licence should be developed to the full. At the same time, they stressed most strongly that 'the real criterion of deficiency is a social one'. The distinction between the patient in hospital and the patient under voluntary supervision had nothing to do with his scholastic ability. It depended entirely on whether he was capable of living a normal life under reasonably sheltered conditions without being exploited by other people, or himself causing difficulty in his environment. Those who were anti-social or in moral danger (such as alcoholics and over-sexed young women) would continue to need institutional care; but the quiet, stable kind of defective, even with a comparatively low intelligence, might be discharged to the care of a suitable social worker.

Institutional Care

In a memorable phrase, the Wood Committee laid down that the mental deficiency institution should be 'not a stagnant pool, but a flowing lake'. It should be equipped with a school, workshops, playing-fields and a small hospital block—the general outline being closer to that of a boarding-school than to that of a hospital; and the object should be to prepare patients for life in the community—not simply to confine them for life. The work of the 'school' would include much that elsewhere might be termed occupational therapy or even physio-therapy. Some patients would have to be taught the primary co-ordination of muscles—how to walk, how to climb stairs, and so on—while others could progress to simple handwork. Some might also be taught the normal primary school subjects, and older patients would learn simple processes in the workshops.

The Committe thought that the defective's failure to make a social response was often due to the fact that he could not work, and was thus dependent on charity. 'To deal with a defective simply as a pauper is to ostracize him: but let him render the community some service, however modest or humble, and he will acquire some measure of self-respect, and thus take the initial step towards socialization.'

It suggested also the extension of the 'half-way house' principle. A few authorities had already acquired hostels where suitable defectives could live under supervision while going out to work each day. The cost of maintenance was low, because the defectives could contribute towards their keep, or even pay the whole cost of it; and the patients had a greater degree of freedom and normality in living than was possible in the institution proper.

Main Recommendations

The chief conclusions reached by the Wood Committee after its five years of deliberation were these:

1. The real criterion of mental deficiency should be social inefficiency, not educational subnormality.
2. The powers and duties of local mental deficiency authorities should be widened to deal with all mental defectives except those between five and fifteen who were capable of attending special schools run by the education authority.
3. The Board of Control should continue to be directly responsible for the management of institutions for those with 'incorrigible criminal tendencies'.[1]
4. Greater use should be made of all forms of community care—licensing from institutions, half-way houses, guardianship, statutory and voluntary supervision.
5. There should ultimately be a co-ordinated mental health service—one local authority in each area responsible for both mental patients and mental defectives. A specialist mental health officer should serve on the staff of the local health authority to co-ordinate and supervise this work.

The Local Government Act of 1929, which broke up the old Poor Law framework, made possible the transfer of certain Poor Law institutions to the mental deficiency authorities, and also provided for the transfer of responsibility for defectives receiving out-relief. The other recommendations—with the exception of the last, which was not to be implemented until the passing of the National Health Service Act seventeen years later—were a matter of departmental arrangement, and of reorientation of attitudes in dealing with mental defectives.

The growth of the community services for defectives which followed the circulation of this report was considerable. In 1929, the total number of persons cared for by mental deficiency authorities—including those in institutions—was 40,000. By 1934, the figures for community care alone were as follows:

[1] Moss Side and Rampton institutions for defectives of this type had been founded after the First World War. There was also Broadmoor, founded in 1864, and at this time under the jurisdiction of the Home Office.

Guardianship	. .	3,083
Stat. supervision	. .	33,377
Vol. supervision	. .	22,544

59,004

By this time, thirteen hospitals were sending patients out to daily work; nine hostels were in operation; and the number of occupation and industrial centres had risen to 191.[1]

REPORT OF THE BROCK COMMITTEE 1934

The Wood Committee, in its report, had made a courageous effort to deal with the question of mental deficiency as a genetic and social problem. This was still a highly controversial field where few facts were definitely established. The Wood Committee drew a distinction between primary amentia—due to germinal variation or defect—and secondary amentia—due to some accident or condition affecting a foetus or a live child. Primary amentia they described as 'the last stage of the inheritance of degeneracy of the subnormal group'. This subnormal group represented the lowest tenth of the population measured in social efficiency—the insane, the paupers, the epileptics, the criminals, the alcoholics, the prostitutes and the unemployables. They saw only two methods by which the existence of this sub-normal group could be eliminated—segregation and sterilization. It was essential that the 'lowest tenth' should be prevented from propagating its own kind.

Secondary amentia was a different matter. Here the inheritance was sound, and the causes of deterioration or destruction of brain tissue could be dealt with individually. Secondary amentia might be pre-natal—caused by an alcoholic or a syphilitic condition in the mother, for example. It might be natal—due to injuries from instruments or natural causes during the process of birth; or it might be post-natal. Cretinism was already recognized as a condition due to thyroid deficiency, and treatable by medical means. Similarly, treatments were being evolved for the hypo- and hyper-pituitary conditions. There was good hope that secondary amentia could gradually be eliminated by improvements in surgical and medical techniques.

Primary amentia remained the problem. Segregation was efficient, but very costly; and it turned the mental deficiency institution into a

[1] Annual Report of the Board of Control, 1934.

place of detention rather than a hospital. Sterilization was a highly controversial matter, involving religious and ethical principles as well as considerations of practicability.

At that time, twenty-two American States had sterilization laws, but only two had enforced them on any considerable scale. Even in these two states, it had not been found that the practice of sterilization noticeably reduced the numbers of mental defectives requiring institutional treatment. There were so many other factors besides that of propagation, which might render a defective incapable of normal living.

The practical argument against sterilization was that it would make doctors even more reluctant to certify a patient as a mental defective than they already were; and therefore that it might materially hinder the work of ascertainment. The medical argument was that both diagnosis and prognosis were extremely difficult, and that there would be great difficulty in making such an irrevocable decision in any particular case. From the psychological point of view, sterilization might have disastrous effects on the patient's personality, involving a deep and lasting loss of self-respect. From a religious stand-point, it involved depriving human beings of a fundamental human right—that of reproduction.

Yet, when all these arguments had been put forward, the fact remained that this group, the 'submerged tenth', was widely recognized; and that there seemed no other way of preventing it from growing and from being a permanent drag on the rest of the community.

In 1934, a departmental committee was set up under the chairmanship of L. G. (later Sir Laurence) Brock, Chairman of the Board of Control,[1] to investigate the question of legal sterilization. On behalf of the Committee, Dr. Lionel Penrose and Dr. Douglas Turner, two authorities on mental deficiency work, made an investigation through the agency of the local education authorities. They found that, of the children of mental defectives between the ages of seven and thirteen, 40·4 per cent were either mentally defective or seriously retarded. Of these, they considered that rather less than a third were definitely primary aments.

The evidence that primary amentia existed on a wide scale was there; but it was not so wide-spread as to justify sterilization at all costs. The Brock Committee concluded that sterilization should be legalized; but that it should be on a voluntary basis only, and subject to stringent safeguards.

[1] 1879–1949. Formerly Assistant Secretary to the Ministry of Health.

Persons who might apply for sterilization were:

  (i) mental defectives;
 (ii) the mentally disordered;
(iii) those suffering from grave physical defects which had been shown to be transmissible;
 (iv) mental 'carriers', i.e. those who, while not suffering from mental disorder or defect themselves in an appreciable degree, had such a morbid heredity that they might produce mentally unfit children.

The legal safeguards were first, the necessity for the free consent of the patient; second, a recommendation from two independent medical practitioners; and third, the approval in each individual case of the Ministry of Health.

This was a curious report. Mental defectives and certified mental patients were by definition people who were incapable of clear volition on major issues. To expect them to make a decision of such magnitude, involving consequences which they could not fully appreciate, was asking a great deal. The number of those suffering from major physical defects which could be proved to be transmissible (such as certain kinds of deaf mutism and blindness) was probably very small; and the definition of a mental 'carrier' and 'morbid inheritance' was going to be very difficult indeed. Doctors and social workers could bring forward individual cases where sterilization seemed a clear necessity, and where the patient's consent could be obtained without undue influence being brought to bear; but to frame a law which would cover these cases while not leaving any loophole for abuse was another matter. American experience showed that even when the law was on the Statute Book, public opinion could kill it.

The Minister of Health, Sir Hilton Young, walked carefully. He was 'profoundly impressed by the strength of the reasons given by the Committee in support of their recommendations' and, as far as his own individual conscience was concerned, could see no difficulty in giving them his full approval. As a Minister of the Crown, however, he held a wider responsibility. 'We must remember that this is a novel question, and one which has not yet been thought out by the mind and heart of the nation. At the present time, consideration is being given to the report by the great organizations of national opinion, such as the Churches. I think it would be wrong from a ministerial point of view to propose any national policy in the matter until there has been sufficient time for the national mind and conscience to be cleared. . . .'[1]

---

[1] *Hansard*, June 20th, 1934.

Only two Members of Parliament were ready to comment on the Report in the House. One gains the impression that this was such a difficult and controversial issue that the average member was unwilling to say anything which might bring down on him the wrath of his constituents. Wing-Commander James,[1] believed that public opinion was in favour of sterilization, and called for immediate action. Dr. W. J. O'Donovan[2] took the opposite view. In a pungent speech, he called sterilization 'A short-cut method for the surgical relief of poverty' and stated, 'The dullards are as much the dough of society as the brilliant people are the currants . . . there are limits set to the power of the State over the minds and body [*sic*] of men.'

There the Brock Report rested. It had to some extent clarified the situation; but no attempt was made, or has been since, to carry its recommendations into effect. Recent genetic research has modified the view of heredity on which it was based, while the practical and ethical objections have not lost their force. Belief in the hopelessness of the condition of the 'submerged tenth' has been modified by social work practice in the intervening years.

[1] M.P. for Wellingborough, now Sir Archibald James.
[2] A Harley Street specialist in skin disorders.

PART THREE
The Mentally Ill

Chapter Six

THE RESULTS OF LEGALISM

FROM a medical point of view, the Lunacy Act of 1890 was out of date before it was passed. It represented the legal view of mental illness—that here was a condition which made it necessary in certain circumstances to deprive a man of his personal liberty, and that every possible device must be used to limit these circumstances.

Asylums could only take certified patients; and patients could not be certified until the illness had reached a stage where it was obvious to a lay authority—the justice of the peace. This made it impossible for the asylums to deal with early diagnosis, and the treatment of most mild or acute cases. Their work thus became largely custodial.

The difficulties did not end there. Because certification was a necessary preliminary, many doctors tried to avoid sending patients to asylums except as a last resort, and sought other means of treatment;[1] and doctors who wished to specialize in psychiatry often avoided a sphere where most of the work was routine, and where there was little opportunity for improvement of professional techniques.

When new theories of the aetiology of mental illness developed, and new techniques for treatment were formulated, they at first by-passed the asylums completely. The treatment of neurosis developed in the consulting-rooms and the out-patient clinics of the nineteen-twenties and thirties. Later there were new neurosis units, of which the Maudsley was the prototype; but not until after 1930, when the Mental Treatment Act at last presented a means of dealing with mental patients under in-patient conditions without certification, was all this work brought into relation with the asylum service.[2]

[1] Dr. Walk comments, 'The registered hospitals and licensed houses did a brisk trade in recoverable cases.'

[2] See p. 120.

The Decline of Asylum Standards

The barrier of certification and the emphasis on custodialism which resulted from the 1890 Lunacy Act undoubtedly contributed to the decline in standards of care and treatment; but there were other factors involved also. One was the question of size. The original county asylums were small institutions in which it was possible to preserve some of the values of face-to-face relationships. Lincoln Asylum, built in 1820, had only fifty beds. Nottingham (1811) had eighty. Of the first nine asylums, built by 1827, the average size was 116 beds; but almost at once, it became clear that the number of beds needed had been seriously under-estimated in most areas, and the asylums grew rapidly in size. At Lancaster, the asylum was originally constructed in 1816 for 170 patients, and accommodated 600 by 1842. By 1870, the average size in England and Wales was 542 beds; by 1900, it was 961; and by 1930, it was 1,221.[1]

These barrack-like institutions had a very different atmosphere from the small homely asylums of earlier years. With more than ten times as many patients, they were forced to deal with people in the mass. Ten nurses dealing with a ward of a hundred patients do not generally achieve the same quality of personal relationship as one nurse with ten patients—they tend to form a social group of their own. Five doctors dealing with a thousand patients do not exert the same kind of individual influence that one doctor does in a community of two hundred. There was a loss of the sense of community, a quality of de-personalization, which often led to the isolation of the individual patient in a crowd rather than his integration in a friendly group.

Dr. Grenville, in the Report of the *Lancet* Commission, had noted this tendency in 1877. By that date, the number of patients in Hanwell had risen from the original 1,000 to nearly 2,000. 'The treatment,' he wrote, 'is humane, but it necessarily lacks individuality, and that special character which arises from dealing with a limited number of cases directly . . . it is only in a small asylum that this potent remedy, the sane will working quietly, patiently and directly, can be brought to bear on individual cases.'[2]

The medical superintendent was now bound to a heavy burden of paper-work which involved the repeated notification of details concerning every individual case to a central authority in London. Though

[1] See Appendix II.
[2] Op. cit., vol. I, pp. 81, 254.

other doctors might be employed on the asylum staff, the full responsibility for fulfilling the requirements of the law was his; but the requirements of the law were primarily concerned with ensuring that patients had been rightfully deprived of their personal liberty—not with what happened to them afterwards. In these circumstances, it is scarcely surprising that the gentle permissive influence which had characterized the best of the early asylums could no longer flourish.

The architecture of the asylums built in the late nineteenth century is indicative of the theory of mental illness which lay behind their building. Long corridors, large square wards and stout lockable doors made for easy surveillance. Patients worked on the farms and gardens, in the laundries and sewing-rooms; but their work was organized for the maintenance of the institution, not for their own benefit. They moved from place to place in groups, and they were 'counted in' and 'counted out' of the ward by nurses who often could not remember names or faces.

The Impact of the First World War

War was to reduce standards of staffing and accommodation still further. The second Annual Report of the Board of Control (1915) stated that 42 per cent of asylum medical staff had volunteered, and been accepted, for military service. A special mention was made of Dr. Crowther, newly-appointed medical superintendent of Netherne Hospital. On appointment, he asked that he might be allowed to defer taking up his duties until the end of the war; and the retiring superintendent, who had reached pensionable age, agreed to remain in office for that period. Dr. Crowther enlisted for combatant service, became a despatch rider, and was killed by a shell at Armentières only a few weeks later. With varying degrees of tragedy, this story was repeated many times. The places of these trained and experienced men were taken by the physically unfit, or by retired medical practitioners with no previous experience of work in this specialist field. The loss to the patients was incalculable.

The Board of Control had no figures on the number of nursing staff who left for active service; but they believed that it was considerably higher than the figure quoted for medical staff. It was often impossible to replace mental nurses, even by untrained workers.

When war broke out, there were 140,466 'notified insane persons' distributed among ninety-seven borough asylums. London had ten asylums, of which eight had more than 2,000 beds. Lancashire had five, all of more than 2,000 beds. Asylums in small towns, on the other hand, often had only 300 or 400 beds. In all areas, there was a degree of over-crowding. By 1915, the position had worsened considerably, since nine of the larger asylums had been placed at the disposal of the War Office as military hospitals. As a result, the remaining mental hospitals became crowded with displaced patients. Standards of both care and treatment suffered.

One odd result of war conditions is that, during the war years, the number of 'notified insane persons' was considerably reduced. The figure for 1915 showed an increase of 2,411 on the previous year; but by the end of that year, the number had been reduced by 3,278. From that time, there was a marked reduction each year until about 1920—when the figures show a return to the pre-war increase rate of 2,000 to 3,000 a year.[1]

There were roughly 2,000 nervous and mental cases in military hos-pitals who would ultimately be certified; but even so, the variation in the annual incidence is sufficiently striking to require some explanation. War brings many kinds of mental stress: fear of death and disablement, grief at the death or disablement of others, bewilderment and rootless-ness and loss of security. It would seem reasonable to expect that, if any variation took place, it would be in the form of an increase in mental illness. One explanation for the decrease is that war intensifies the sense of a communal purpose: that in war-time, everybody is busy, and has a task to fulfill. There is not much time for loneliness, and there are few opportunities for introspection. The stress of poverty is considerably reduced, too, for war usually brings material prosperity. Above all, there is an emotional focus—an enemy to hate, the weak to defend (note the amount of public sentiment poured out at this time on 'Little Belgium') and allies to support. Even grief and fear are not isolating factors, as they often are under normal conditions, for there is a con-sciousness that many others have the same griefs and the same fears. In short, many people suffered stress; but it was a bearable stress, because it was shared.

That is one explanation. It has received considerable support from the medical profession, notably from Professor F. A. E. Crew, late Professor of Social Medicine in the University of Edinburgh, on the grounds that those who are part of a close-knit social group seldom suffer from mental breakdown, and that the strong sense of group participa-

---

[1] Annual Report of the Board of Control, 1915-20. See Appendix I. A similar situation arose in the Second World War. See p. 143.

tion is a significant factor in the reduction of mental illness observable under war conditions.[1] But there is another explanation of a less encouraging nature.

War-time economy establishes an unusual series of priorities. The fitness and efficiency of the men in the Services is a top priority; next comes the well-being of productive workers. The mentally ill come a long way down the scale, for they play no part in the war effort; and their existence is, in fact, a handicap to the purpose in hand. The available beds are overcrowded, there are less doctors and nurses to give treatment, and the general emphasis is on giving treatment only where absolutely necessary. As a result, the decline in the number of those certified in the period 1914–18, may be due, at least in part, not to a decline in the amount of mental illness, but to a reluctance on the part of doctors to certify when adequate treatment was unlikely to follow certification.

Theory and Practice After the War

When the war was over, conditions in the mental hospitals, as they were now increasingly being called, began to improve again. Staff were demobilized, war hospitals closed down, and their premises returned. Members of the Board of Control also returned to normal duty; and in 1918, the Board drafted a report[2] for the Government Reconstruction Committee, making recommendations for the future.

The chief recommendation was that there should be treatment for limited periods without certification. Under the 1890 Act, it was possible for voluntary patients to be admitted to private, but not to public, asylums.[3] A Bill 'to facilitate the early treatment of mental disorder of recent origin' by means of voluntary admission had been introduced into the Commons by Cecil Harmsworth in 1915; but the time had proved unsuitable, and the Bill was withdrawn before the second reading.[4] Now that staffing and accommodation were improving, the proposal was renewed.

Together with this recommendation for the wider provision of voluntary treatment, the Board recommended that general hospitals should develop sections for the early diagnosis and treatment of mental

---

[1] Report of Annual Conference of the National Association of Mental Health, 1955.
[2] Annual Report of the Board of Control, 1918.
[3] With the exception of the Maudsley Hospital. See p. 104.
[4] *Hansard*, April 20th and May 17th, 1915.

illness, both for in- and out-patients. The gap between the treatment of mental and physical illness was imperceptibly narrowing, and it was felt that there should be provision, in the normal scope of the health services, for the many border-line cases.

Third, the Board of Control recommended that the more responsible posts in mental hospitals should be restricted to medical practitioners possessing the Diploma in Psychological Medicine, or Diploma in Mental Diseases, as it was then sometimes termed. This diploma had been instituted in three universities—Edinburgh, Durham and London —in 1911, following a circular letter sent to all universities by the president of the Medico-Psychological Association in 1908-9. This was a parallel development to the institution of specialist post-graduate diplomas in other branches of medicine. By 1918, courses for the D.M.D. were also organized by the Royal College of Physicians, and by the Universities of Leeds and Cambridge.

Fourth, the Board recommended the official encouragement of mental out-patient clinics, which they considered 'inseparably connected with the improvement of methods of dealing with incipient insanity'. These clinics had arisen first in university centres—the Report mentioned Sheffield, Manchester and Birmingham by name—and had excited considerable interest in the medical world.[1]

The fifth and last major recommendation was that the Board of Control should be empowered to make grants for the continuation of after-care work by voluntary societies.

Here we have the essence of the developments of the nineteen-thirties: the extension of voluntary treatment, the narrowing of the gap between mental and physical illness, the development of higher professional standards in psychiatry, out-patient clinics and after-care work; but although the need for these improvements was seen by the Board of Control, they could not be introduced suddenly on a national scale. The number of things that can be achieved by Act of Parliament alone is very small. The Board had to wait for the development of responsible public opinion—of groups which would press for legislative action as the National Association for the Care of the Feeble-Minded had pressed in an allied sphere.

By 1921, any plans for immediate improvement in mental hospital conditions had to be shelved. The Geddes Axe fell, severely curtailing expenditure in all government departments.

---

[1] Some asylums had a small number of out-patients from the eighteen-eighties. This development was not as new as the Board of Control's Report suggested.

The Board reported 'great administrative difficulty. The stringency of the financial conditions prevailing throughout the country had compelled local authorities to check their expenditure in every possible direction'. Hardly any capital expenditure was authorized; and with post-war inflation, maintenance costs had risen considerably.

Thus on the financial side, the picture was a black one. The Board had excellent intentions, but its work was still suffering from the exigencies of the war years; and in a period when money for capital projects was hard to find, there was not a public mandate of sufficient force to demand that money be found.

Administrative Change, 1919

One hopeful augury for the future was the setting-up of the Ministry of Health in 1919. The Local Government Board, which had inherited the powers of the Poor Law Board, and much of its attitude to social misfortune, was finally swept away. There was some significance in the fact that the new authority was entitled the Ministry of Health—public health was no longer to be conceived of as a junior partner to Poor Law administration, concerned only with the health of a section of the population.

The new Ministry' took over all the functions of the Local Government Board, including the responsibility for many matters only indirectly connected with health policy, such as Poor Law, Housing and Local Government.

Within a year of its inception, the Ministry of Health took over powers in the control of lunacy and mental deficiency. By the Ministry of Health (Lunacy and Mental Deficiency, Transfer of Powers) Order,[1] it assumed those powers which were given to the Home Office under the Mental Deficiency Act of 1913. These included the general power to make regulations determining the activities of the Board of Control (section 25); the supervision and regulation of the activities of local authorities (section 30); the right to appoint the chairman of the Board of Control (section 22, iii) and the right to appoint and fix the salaries of the Board's secretary and inspectors (section 23, ii).

The Board of Control, though it imperceptibly lost its quasi-independent status after the acquisition of this new and powerful overseer, welcomed the change as 'an important step towards bringing the Board of Control into a proper and desirable relation with the central

[1] S.R. and O. 1920. No. 809.

health authority'. The way was now open for the ultimate assimilation of the treatment of mental illness with that of physical illness.

The Prestwich Enquiry

One of the smaller powers affected by the Transfer of Powers Order of 1920 was that which enabled the Ministry to hold a public enquiry if the Board reported that a local authority was thought not to be carrying out its duties under the Lunacy and Mental Deficiency Acts. Within two years, this power was to be used by the Minister of Health in an enquiry at Prestwitch Hospital, Manchester.

From 1922, there began the growth of a public interest in this field which can be compared more easily with the three 'waves of suspicion and excitement' of the nineteenth century,[1] than with any more recent development. The agitation started with a book about Prestwich Hospital—*The Experiences of an Asylum Doctor*, written by Dr. Montague Lomax, and published soon after the end of the war.

The picture which Dr. Lomax drew was a grim one. He stated that the patients were poorly fed and poorly clad; that they were closely confined, though a number of them would have benefited from parole, with no detriment to the community; that the nurses were mostly unqualified, unsuited to the nature of their work, and that they had, in a number of specific cases, treated the patients with open cruelty. It was a picture of a drab institution life, unrelieved by hope or sympathy or understanding, where, as a result largely of ignorance and neglect, appalling cruelties were still possible.

The Minister of Health was then Alfred Mond; and when a spate of newspaper articles and indignant speeches followed the book's publication, he appointed a committee of the Ministry of Health 'to enquire into the administration of Public Mental Hospitals'. Being a departmental committee, it was responsible directly to the Minister, and not to Parliament. It had the advantage of being a small committee, and therefore of being able to report more speedily. The members were Sir Cyril Cobb, M.P.;[2] Dr. R. Percy Smith;[3] and Dr. Bedford Pierce.[4] Their task was to enquire first, whether Dr. Lomax had given a faithful representation of conditions at Prestwich; and second, whether his

---

[1] See D. H. Tuke's description in *Chapters in the History of the Insane*, p. 190.

[2] M.P. for W. Fulham. A barrister and formerly chairman of the L.C.C.

[3] Consulting Physician for Mental Disorders, St. Thomas's Hospital.

[4] Lecturer in Mental Disorders, University of Leeds. A former medical superintendent of the Retreat.

charges were applicable to other mental hospitals. The three members of the Committee visited the hospital, and undertook a personal enquiry.

They pointed out in their Report that Dr. Lomax had served in Prestwich during the war, when conditions were far from typical. Moreover, he had no special qualification in psychiatry, and might therefore misconstrue certain measures of policy. They found no actual evidence of cruelty or flagrant abuse, and considered the part of the book relating to these charges to be unfounded.

At the same time, they agreed that conditions at Prestwich were not good. There was a great lack of staff, particularly trained staff; and a number of unsuitable untrained staff had had to be recruited, in order to keep the institution running at all. Lack of suitable staff led to a severe curtailment of the activities of the hospital. Thus it was seldom possible to allow patients out of the building, because there were no nurses who could be freed from other duties to accompany them. They agreed that the patients were poorly and uniformly clothed, and that their diet was monotonous and unappetizing.

How far did these considerations apply to other mental hospitals? The Committee was greatly hampered in its work of discovery by the fact that, being only a departmental committee, it had no power to hear witnesses on oath, or to protect them against subsequent victimization. The Asylum Workers' Union, a body whose views on this subject should have been heard, refused to give evidence, or to allow its members to do so in an individual capacity, for this reason.[1] There seems little doubt now that the conclusions of the Committee were tempered by the partial nature of the evidence available to them.

The Committee accordingly had to confine their general findings to two major considerations: the construction of mental hospitals, and the recruitment of staff. They deprecated the erection of large barrack-like hospitals of the Prestwich type, and recommended that future mental hospitals should not have more than one thousand beds. They recommended construction on the villa-system, a number of small, separate units of accommodation being spread round the grounds.[2] This would make possible the designation of separate reception and convalescent wards, so that those patients who were most in contact with the community outside could be kept away from the 'asylum' atmosphere. They thought also that it was unwise to mix patients from differing

---

[1] The A.W.U. did give evidence before the Royal Commission two years later.

[2] Some hospitals had built villa-units in the 1880's and after; but the Committee's recommendation referred to the construction of the entire hospital.

social backgrounds—'some account should be taken of home conditions and the surroundings from which the patient has come'.

As far as the staffing situation was concerned, the Committee found that in general there was a great lack of suitable nursing staff, both male and female. This was of course nothing new—for there had never been enough of the right kind of people to take up this exacting and widely misunderstood type of work; but the situation had been aggravated by the war. In 1922, the conversion from war to peace economy was not yet fully completed, and there was no real shortage of more congenial employment for those who sought it.

Examinations for nurses had been started on a national scale by the Royal Medico-Psychological Association in 1891.

In 1919, the Nurses' Registration Act made provisions for state registration, and for the setting up of the General Nursing Council. The G.N.C. refused to recognize the existing R.M.P.A. examinations for mental nurses, stating that, as a matter of policy, it intended to run its own examinations and not to recognize the results of any other body. The Mental Nursing Certificate of the G.N.C. was instituted in 1921. The theoretical standard required was higher than that of the R.M.P.A. examination.

By 1922, then, there were two separate forms of qualification for mental nurses; and there were many mental nurses with neither the will nor the apparent ability to take either. Prestwich was not alone in this respect.

Chapter Seven

INTO THE COMMUNITY

WHILE the position in the asylums was a depressing one, and the work of the Board of Control and the more enlightened and devoted staff seemed to bring little progress, movements outside the normal administrative structure offered much hope for the future. Of these, perhaps the most far-reaching were the opening of the Maudsley Hospital to voluntary patients in 1923, and the growth of the Mental After-Care Association.

The Maudsley Hospital

Dr. Henry Maudsley, who was a son-in-law of John Conolly, had a brilliant career in psychiatry, and his personal influence was a major factor in the growth of this specialism in medicine.[1] Medical superintendent of the Manchester Royal Lunatic Hospital[2] at the age of twenty-three, he followed Dr. Bucknill as editor of the *Journal of Mental Science*. In 1869 he became Professor of Medical Jurisprudence at University College Hospital, London, where Conolly himself had held a Chair for a time. In 1907, he decided on a generous and practical way of giving expression to his own ideas and those of his colleagues, on mental treatment.[3] He offered £30,000 to the London County Council for a new mental hospital, on three conditions: it was to deal exclusively with early and acute cases; it was to have an out-patients' clinic; and it

[1] 1835–1918. *Who's Who*, 1917 and *Annual Register*, 1918. Surprisingly, no account of his life is given in D.N.B.

[2] Founded in 1763 as a branch of the Infirmary at Manchester; now Cheadle Royal Hospital.

[3] A movement for a 'psychiatric clinic' of this nature had been discussed among psychiatrists for some twenty years before this date.

was to provide for teaching and research on the diagnosis and treatment of mental disorder.

The London County Council accepted this offer, and the new hospital was built at a total cost of over a quarter of a million pounds.[1] It was completed in 1915, in which year parliamentary sanction was secured to enable it to take patients without certification under the 1890 Act, thus anticipating the Mental Treatment Act of 1930 by fifteen years.[2] From 1915 until the end of the war, it was used as a war hospital, and the Ministry of Pensions continued to use it for the treatment of shell-shock cases until 1923. In that year, the Maudsley reverted to its original purpose.[3]

The classification and treatment of the neuroses, which owed much to the work of the psycho-analytic school, notably Kraepelin and Freud, had become a matter of urgent public interest as a result of the war. Cases of 'shell-shock'—the Second World War was to produce the term 'battle fatigue' for the same condition—had swamped the military hospitals. There was a gradual recognition that this was a form of mental illness, which, though not amounting to what was then termed insanity, was seriously disabling, but susceptible to treatment. The Maudsley had already pioneered in the treatment of war cases. From 1923, it was free to deal also with the neuroses of a peace-time economy, which, though sometimes less dramatic in form, were no less seriously disabling.

In 1924, the Maudsley became a teaching school of the University of London—the first in the psychiatric field. In 1936, Chairs in Psychiatry and in the Pathology of Mental Disease were instituted. The London County Council continued to bear the full cost of this undertaking until 1946, when, after an inter-departmental committee on medical schools had pointed out that the hospital occupied 'a special place in psychiatric work' and was serving a national purpose, the financial burden was taken over by the University of London.

The influence of the Maudsley as a centre of teaching and research has been incalculable. It received due recognition on the inception of the National Health Service in 1948 when, united with Bethlem, England's oldest mental hospital, it was designated as the only post-graduate teaching hospital exclusive to psychiatry. The medical school was then renamed the Institute of Psychiatry, and became one of the constituent institutes of the British Post-graduate Medical Federation.

---

[1] Dr. Maudsley subsequently increased his donation by £10,000.
[2] Under the L.C.C. (parks, etc.). Act of 1915.
[3] K. J. Johnson, 'Bethlem and the Maudsley', *Bethlem and Maudsley Gazette*.

The Mental After-Care Association

Though the major part in progress in the care of the mentally ill was played by statutory organizations, voluntary agencies had begun to play a part in this field also. The earliest of these was the Mental After-Care Association, founded in 1879. The impetus for the foundation of this society came from the chaplain of the Middlesex Asylum at Colney Hatch, who published two papers on social after-care in the *Journal of Mental Science*.[1] In these papers, he stressed the urgent necessity for some intermediate form of care for discharged mental patients. 'The prospect of permanent recovery,' he pointed out, 'greatly depends on the patient's circumstances on first resuming life's ordinary associations.' He pleaded for 'a brief interval of seasonable repose' for the patient facing the complexities and pitfalls of life in the community.

These papers aroused a wide-spread interest, and in June, 1879, a meeting took place in Dr. Bucknill's house[2] in Wimpole Street at which the chaplain, Mr. Hawkins, and several leading alienists were present. Among them was Dr. Hack Tuke.[3] An association was formed, Dr. Bucknill becoming the first president, and Mr. Hawkins the secretary. In 1880, the Earl of Shaftesbury, chairman of the Lunacy Commissioners, accepted an offer of the presidency. He expressed his conviction that 'The After-Care Association was required to supply a real want. It was a seed plot from which in time good results would spring'.[4]

The work of the Association was on a comparatively small scale. As Madeline Rooff comments, 'The propaganda of this small society was very gentle, and its work in community care proceeded patiently and slowly in the early years of the twentieth century.'[5] The number of cases dealt with in 1887 was 41. In 1900, it had risen to 195, and in 1918 to 670. By this time, its finances were stretched to the limit. The work carried out was of two kinds, residential and personal. Residental after-care took the form of placing ex-patients for a short period in convalescent homes run by ex-matrons or senior nursing officers from the asylums, and paying a maintenance charge for them. Patients were sometimes also boarded out with individual families. Personal after-

[1] Rev. H. Hawkins, *A Plea for Convalescent Homes in connection with Asylums for the Insane Poor*, 1871 and *After Care*, 1879.
[2] 39, Wimpole Street. For Dr. Bucknill, see p. 13n.
[3] See p. 14.
[4] Presidential address, 1883, quoted in M.A.C.A. leaflet.
[5] M. Rooff, *Voluntary Societies and Social Policy*, p. 95.

care was carried out by a number of 'voluntary associates', who undertook this work as a form of charitable enterprise. They found work and lodgings for friendless patients, or sometimes helped to adjust difficult family situations.

In 1919, M.A.C.A.'s work was recognized and considerably increased when the London County Council Asylums and Mental Deficiency Department authorized its sub-committees to make use of the Association in dealing with patients discharged on trial, and to make payments up to the full cost of maintenance.

By 1924, the Association was handling a fair amount of early care and after-care work in the London area.[1] Its pioneer work, in close connection with the statutory authorities, was repeatedly commended by the Board of Control in its Annual Reports, and was one of the factors considered by the Royal Commission of 1924–6 in its survey of the whole field of the care of mental patients.

THE ROYAL COMMISSION OF 1924-6

On July 25th, 1924, a Royal Commission on Lunacy and Mental Disorder was appointed. From the Board of Control's comments in their report for that year, it appears that the immediate cause of the appointment of the Commission was not its own desire to achieve legislation of a more enlightened type, but the 'uneasiness aroused in the public mind by a number of charges, somewhat recklessly made, to the effect that large numbers of sane persons were being detained as insane, that the whole system of lunacy administration was wrong, and that widespread cruelty existed in our public mental hospitals'.

The Commission's terms of reference, however, were wide enough to secure constructive as well as destructive evidence. They were to enquire into 'the existing law and administrative machinery in England and Wales in connection with the certification detention and care of persons who are, or who are alleged to be of unsound mind' and also into 'the extent to which provision is or should be made ... for the treatment without certification of persons suffering from mental disorder'. They were not to deal with mental deficiency or with criminal lunacy.

The Royal Commission was appointed by the Home Secretary, the

[1] A branch was formed in Birmingham in 1912, but there was otherwise little activity in the provinces. 1,176 cases were dealt with in the London area in this year.

Rt. Hon. Arthur Henderson. The majority of its members had legal qualifications—the chairman, Hugh Pattison (later Lord) Macmillan, was the Lord Advocate for Scotland. Other members included the future Lord Jowitt, then a K.C., and Member of Parliament for West Hartlepool; Sir Ernest Hiley, a solictor who had been Town Clerk successively of Leicester and Birmingham; F. D. (later Lord) Mackinnon, who was to resign early in the Commission's proceedings on his appointment as a High Court judge; the second Earl Russell, grandson of Lord John Russell, and elder brother of Bertrand Russell, who was a barrister; Sir Thomas Hutchinson, recently Lord Provost of Edinburgh; and Nathaniel Micklem, K.C., who had retired from practice in the previous year.

There were two medical members—Sir Humphrey Rolleston and Sir David Drummond. Both possessed legal as well as medical qualifications. Sir Humphrey was at that time president of the Royal College of Physicians—a practising physician whose major interest lay in organic diseases and the physical decay associated with old age. Sir David was Professor of Medicine in the University of Durham, and an authority on diseases of the brain and the nervous system.

Two Members of Parliament were appointed—in addition to Jowitt, whose interest was primarily a legal one. They were Lord Eustace Percy, a younger son of the Duke of Northumberland, and Mr. Harry Snell. Lord Eustace, whose major interests lay in the field of education and public administration, resigned late in 1924 on his appointment as president of the Board of Education. Thirty years later, he was to return to this subject as chairman of the Royal Commission on Mental Illness and Mental Deficiency appointed in 1954. Mr. Snell was a Labour member with a background of Co-operative and Trade Union interests, and became one of the first Labour peers in 1931.

The Commission set out to do two things: it received evidence on the existing system from those who operated it—Government departments, voluntary agencies, Relieving Officers, magistrates, psychiatrists and others; then it turned to receive evidence on the shortcomings of the existing system from the National Society for Lunacy Reform and from individual members of the public. Here there is some evidence of impatience among the Committee's members. The National Society for Lunacy Reform brought forward a number of ex-patients who wished to give evidence. After the first day's hearing in public, the Commission decided that the atmosphere was one of 'recrimination and controversy', and directed that future hearings of this kind should be held in camera. 'We do not find,' they record, 'that the evidence received from this source made any constructive contribution to the main purpose of our Inquiry.'[1] Again, the Commission received over 360 letters from patients. 'Some of these,' they note, 'were unintelligible.' These letters were presumably passed on the Board of Control, but it is perhaps an indication of the growing remoteness of twentieth-century administration that very little time could be spared for the investigation of individual cases, and that almost all of the evidence came from official and semi-official sources. In the past, agencies with an exclusively 'liberty-of-the-subject' interest had often been clamorous, time-wasting and retrogressive. Nevertheless, this kind of agitation was an outlet for a genuine public anxiety, and might have been allowed a greater measure of publicity.

The Existing System

The Commission found that there still existed a clear distinction between the treatment of paupers and that of persons of means. In this respect, 'pauper' had a special meaning, since it referred to any patient maintained in a public asylum, even though the relatives were in fact paying the whole cost of maintenance. Because they could not afford private treatment, the old connection with the Poor Law remained. Admission procedure was by the 'observation' order (1890 Act, sections 20 and 21) and the summary reception order (sections 13–19). The 'observation' order had an initial duration of three days, but could be extended for a further fourteen. It involved the removal of a patient by a police constable or a Relieving Officer to a workhouse until suitable provision for treatment could be made.[2] The summary reception order required that proceedings should be taken by the Relieving Officer, and that there should be one medical certificate and a magistrate's order. These procedures, which brought upon the family the double stigma of insanity and Poor Law, were often a source of much distress, and therefore a barrier to early treatment.

For a person of means, it was still possible to obtain a writ from a Judge in Lunacy *de lunatico inquirendo*.[3] This procedure was still relatively costly, and its use was rare. The usual methods of certification were the urgency order and the order on petition. Under the 1890 Act,

[1] This evidence was published among the minutes of the Royal Commission.
[2] This might in some cases be a special ward or block reserved for these patients.
[3] See K. Jones, *Lunacy, Law, and Conscience, 1744–1845*, pp. 221–3.

an urgency order (section ii) had a duration of only seven days, and was obtainable on the application of a relative and one medical certificate. An order on petition (sections 4–8) required a relative's application, a magistrate's order, and two medical certificates.

Private patients were still to be found in licensed houses, registered hospitals, single care (which classification might include treatment in a nursing home if the patient were the only mental patient in that particular home) and in amenity beds in the public mental hospitals. 'Pauper' patients were accommodated generally in the public mental hospitals, though a proportion—the Report did not state how many—were still in Poor Law institutions.

General Considerations of Policy

(i) *The interaction of mental and physical illness.* Perhaps the most valuable part of the Commission's work, from a long-term viewpoint, lay in its statements on the nature of mental illness. They are the product of expert knowledge and clear-thinking—a fairly rare combination in mental health work at this time.

Mental illness was defined as 'the inability of the patient to maintain his social equilibrium'. This was 'essentially a public health problem, to be dealt with on modern public health lines'. It should be a community service, based on the treatment of patients in their own homes wherever possible, and with a strong preventive element.

The statement on the interaction of mental and physical illness has become a classic, and is here quoted in full:

'It has become increasingly evident that there is no clear line of demarcation between mental and physical illness. The distinction as commonly drawn is based on a difference of symptoms. In ordinary parlance, a disease is described as mental if its symptoms manifest themselves predominantly in derangement of conduct, and as physical if its symptoms manifest themselves predominantly in derangement of bodily function. A mental illness may have physical concomitants; probably it always has, though they may be difficult of detection. A physical illness, on the other hand, may have, and probably always has, mental concomitants. And there are many cases in which it is a question whether the physical or the mental symptoms predominate.'

This was perhaps a common-place to psychiatrists; but for many people, even in the medical profession, it was thinking of a new kind.

Insanity had always been treated as a subject bearing little relation to general medicine. This statement, backed by two of the greatest medical brains of the day, meant that a patient should no longer be regarded as a 'case' of peptic ulcer or dermatitis, schizophrenia or hysteria. He was a unique fusion of mind and body, and illness, whether mental or physical in symptomatology, was something which affected his whole nature.

To the psychiatrist, this was not new. Freud had demonstrated long before how many apparent physical ailments could be the product of hysteria, and something was known about the effect of mental processes on skin conditions and gastric disorders; but the authority of this statement, and the wide publicity accorded to it, make it a landmark in the development of the public attitude to mental illness.

(*ii*) *Voluntary treatment.* 'The keynote of the past,' said the Commission, 'has been detention. The keynote of the future should be prevention and treatment.'

The 1890 Act represented one solution to the problem of how to deal with those whose behaviour conflicted with that of the society in which they lived. It was the solution of compulsion, hedged in with 'anxious provisions' and 'bristling with precautions against illegal detention'.

The other solution was voluntary treatment. It had been suggested many years before by Shaftesbury and his associates. It had been granted a grudging and very limited approval in 1862 and 1890 by the provision that voluntary boarders could be accepted in private asylums. It had been pressed for strongly by the Board of Control in 1918. The Maudsley Hospital was the only public hospital where psychiatric in-patient treatment could be given without preliminary certification.[1] The experience of the Maudsley, at that time treating approximately 650 new cases a year, showed that treatment of this kind could be of the greatest benefit to the patient without being in any way a threat to the liberty of the subject. It was especially valuable for the neurotic patient, who was capable of expressing volition and of co-operating in treatment. To certify such a patient was often to destroy the possibility of co-operation.

In other mental hospitals, the old dilemma remained. In order to get treatment, the patient had to be certifiable; and in order to be certifiable, he must have reached such a stage in his illness that he was quite probably incurable. This was 'contrary to the accepted canons of preventive medicine'. Elaborate machinery and legal formalities were posi-

---

[1] There were also a few beds of this kind in the City of London Hospital.

tively harmful. (It should be noted also that the possibility of illegal detention was by this time very small indeed. Licensed houses had greatly decreased in numbers, and those that remained were systematically visited. Mental hospitals were so overcrowded that it is difficult to imagine any medical superintendent keeping patients under detention any longer than was necessary.)

The Commission thought that in future, legal intervention should be confined to three functions: protecting the patient against neglect or ill-treatment; ensuring that his liberty was infringed only as long as necessary in his own or the public interest; and ensuring that he received proper treatment.

(iii) *Class distinctions.* 'The present legal status of the great bulk of insane persons in this country,' noted the Commission, 'is that of paupers'. The Commission recommended not only the abolition of the old connection with the Poor Law, but also the abolition of all legal distinctions between private and pauper patients—'the justification for which has largely disappeared under modern social conditions'. This was a sweeping proposal.

(iv) *Community care.* The Commission felt that much of the good work being done by mental hospitals was being nullified by the lack of suitable help for the patient in the period immediately following discharge. 'The transition from asylum life to the everyday world is a stage of peculiar difficulty for the recovered patient. The home and family life to which he returns may be unsuitable or unsympathetic; employment may be hard to obtain, and friends may be unable or unwilling to help.'

They mentioned the work of the Mental After-Care Association 'with admiration', but pointed out that its work was largely confined to the London area, and that there was no organized after-care work in the provinces. They considered that, as a matter of principle, public funds should be made available for this work.

Recommendations

From the consideration of general issues, the Commission turned to clear-cut recommendations. These are summarized below:

1. Status and composition of the Board of Control: The Board was to remain under the aegis of the Ministry of Health, but to

preserve its quasi-independent status. To meet criticisms that the Board was 'inaccessible', since its members (fifteen Commissioners had been appointed under the Mental Deficiency Act of 1913) were always on visitation, a smaller Board was recommended. This would consist of four members—a lay chairman, a legal member, a medical member, and a woman. Visitation would be carried out by fifteen Assistant Commissioners, while the members of the Board would generally remain in London for administrative work.

2. Admission to mental hospitals: 'The lunacy code should be recast with a view to securing that the treatment of mental disorder should approximate as nearly to the treatment of physical ailments as is consistent with the special safeguards which are indispensable when the liberty of the subject is infringed.' Certification should be a last resort, not a preliminary to treatment; and where it was necessary, there should be no distinction in the method of certification used for private and 'pauper' patients. Voluntary patients should be able to enter mental hospitals without legal formality, and to discharge themselves on giving seventy-two hours' notice to the authorities.

3. After-care: Local authorities should be encouraged to establish out-patient clinics, to provide observation beds in general hospitals, and to finance after-care work. After-care should remain in the hands of voluntary social agencies, and should not be 'an integral part of the official machinery'.

4. Mental hospital administration: Mental hospitals in future should not exceed a thousand beds, and should be constructed on the villa system. Nurses should be graded according to capability—the best receiving double training in both mental and general nursing, the average nurse being trained in mental nursing, and those who could not reach the required standard of theoretical work forming a separate grade. Entertainment and employment for patients should be developed, and a special officer should be appointed in each hospital to take charge of this work of social rehabilitation. Voluntary unofficial visitors should be encouraged to act as friends of the patients; and a closer touch should be maintained between mental hospitals and general practitioners.

DEVELOPMENTS 1926–30

The Royal Commission's Report marked a complete denial of the principles of 1890, and a development from the earlier and more enlightened principles of 1845. The legal view of mental illness was no longer acceptable. The medical view was fully endorsed; and the social view was encouraged in the clauses relating to rehabilitation and aftercare.

The function of a Royal Commission is to sift out existing ideas on the subject under consideration, and to make recommendations which are in accord with informed and progressive opinion. This the Royal Commission of 1924–6 did brilliantly. The Report was more than an analysis of the existing situation. It was also a stage in development.

In its Annual Report for 1927, the Board of Control made a plea for parliamentary action. Legislation had been postponed for a familiar reason—'pressure of parliamentary business'. 'It is regrettable,' stated the Board, 'that the poorer classes should be denied facilities for treatment which are open to those more fortunately circumstanced.'

Inside the mental hospitals, changes were gradually taking place. In some hospitals, patients were allowed to wear their own clothes if they wished, instead of the drab and depressing garments usually provided. Small articles previously regarded as unnecessary for 'paupers' were now being supplied—nail-brushes, for example, and writing paper and envelopes. In some hospitals, the comparatively new invention of the cinema had been introduced, with beneficial effects. (Four years later, the Board was to deplore the coming of the talking film, on the grounds that silent films of good quality were becoming increasingly difficult to obtain, and that talking films were too complicated and too expensive to be used in mental hospitals! Fortunately, this was only a temporary difficulty.)

Occupational therapy was being introduced in some hospitals, on the Dutch pattern. At Santpoort and Maasoord hospitals in Holland, this activity was highly organized, and had proved of great benefit to patients. The Board of Control stressed in 1927, and in subsequent reports, that patients must not be left to 'deteriorate in wearisome idleness'. Some hospital authorities were taking the view that a patient should only work if his employment was of value to the hospital. This was a wrong view. It was of the greatest importance in the patient's treatment and ultimate cure that he should be occupied and interested when not actually receiving treatment—in fact, occupation and interest were part of the treatment. It did not matter whether the work could be sold for profit, or whether it saved the hospital money. The Board stressed again and again the Royal Commission's recommendation that a 'special officer' should be appointed in each hospital to direct the patients' activities.[1]

Physical methods of treatment were rapidly developing. The Board was convinced that research could produce great advances in treatment, but was pessimistic about the financing of large-scale research projects while the purse-strings were held by local authorities.

Pre-care, after-care, and research: these three topics occur repeatedly in the Board's Annual Reports of the late twenties and the early thirties. 'The successful treatment of mental disorders on modern lines,' stated the 1928 Report, 'is prejudiced by the inability to make adequate provision for the patient except during the relatively acute phase.'

Out-patient clinic work was on the increase; but there was still no system of after-care outside the metropolis. In 1928 came the first recommendation from the Board that a mental hospital should have 'someone analogous to the almoner of a large voluntary hospital', whose task it would be to allay the patient's anxieties about home conditions during treatment, and to help him with employment and domestic difficulties after discharge.

This recommendation was evidently made with developments in the training of psychiatric social workers in mind. In 1926, an appeal had been made to the Commonwealth Fund of America by a number of interested individuals, notably Professor Cyril Burt and Mrs. St. Loe Strachey, who were aware of the work which the Fund had undertaken in training psychiatric social workers in the United States. In response, the Fund's trustees offered to train a small group of English social workers, and the first English psychiatric social workers were thus American-trained.

In 1929, the first English training course was begun in the Social Science department of the London School of Economics. This venture, and the foundation of the London child guidance clinic, where students undertook practical work, were at first also financed by the Commonwealth Fund.[2]

In the administrative field also, there were changes about this time

---

[1] There were no trained occupational therapists in England until 1930. See p. 129.

[2] For an account of the origins and development of psychiatric social work in England, see M. Ashdown and S. C. Brown, *Social Service and Mental Health, passim.*

which would materially affect the future. These resulted from the passing of the Local Government Act, 1929, which finally implemented the recommendations of the Royal Commission on the Poor Laws of 1905–9 by breaking up the Poor Law. In a long-overdue reform, Boards of Guardians were abolished, and Public Assistance Committees of the county and county borough councils took their place. The words 'pauper' and 'Poor Law' were replaced by 'rate-aided person' and 'Public Assistance'. The Public Assistance Committee was to work in close collaboration with the health authorities, through the department of the local Medical Officer of Health.

Section 104 of the Local Government Act provided that the Minister might reduce a local authority's grant if certain services were not maintained to his satisfaction; and section 134 listed these services, including lunacy and mental deficiency services. Section 135 provided that, if any material additional expenditure should be imposed on local authorities, provision should be made for an increased contribution out of monies provided by Parliament.

One effect of this Act was thus to provide a groundwork for the development of community mental health services. The local authority, already responsible for in-patient treatment through its Asylum Committee and for mental deficiency work through its Mental Deficiency Committee, acquired a wider responsibility for the poor person suffering from mental illness. The Poor Law had ceased to exist, and much of the stigma of pauperism had gone with it. In the Mental Treatment Act of the following year, Parliament tackled the stigma of certification.

THE MENTAL TREATMENT BILL OF 1928–30

To some extent, these events overlap. The Mental Treatment Bill was initiated in the House of Lords in November, 1928 by Earl Russell, then Parliamentary Secretary to the Ministry of Transport. If opposition to the Bill's abolition of legal safeguards was to come at all, it would come from the Lords, who had imposed those safeguards in 1890. The choice of Lord Russell as sponsor for the Bill is interesting. He explained in his speech that the introduction of the Bill fell outside his normal parliamentary duties, but that he had a close personal acquaintance with the services for the mentally ill. He had been a member of the Royal Commission of 1924–6, and he had been chairman of the Visiting Committee of Hanwell Asylum for some years.

Lord Russell, a barrister himself, took up the legal issue at the outset:

'A doctor is not that sinister figure which in former times he was represented to be, anxious simply to confine a man in a dungeon for life ... he is treating mental disorder in exactly the same way as he treats any other disease, with a sole view to its cure. When we use such phrases as "the liberty of the subject"—and no one attaches more importance to real liberty of the subject than I do—let us reflect on what the circumstances are. If your daughter has a fever, is she not restrained in bed instead of being allowed to run out into the cold air to die of double pneumonia? You do not invite the justices to do that—you do it as a matter of course ... when the patient has recovered, the patient is grateful for it.'

As always, a speech on this subject sparked off opposition; and, as always, it was emotional opposition. On this occasion,[1] the mouthpiece was Viscount Brentford, who, with a lavish use of such terms as 'asylum' and 'insanity', strove to demonstrate that the dangers of 1859 were still present in 1929. Lord Russell's comment was, 'It rather breaks my heart, at this time of day, to hear this sort of statement.'

Yet, so far had public opinion moved, Lord Russell was forced to defend his position from the opposite angle—to defend the retention of a very small degree of legal intervention from those who wanted to sweep it away completely. The clause requiring a voluntary patient to give seventy-two hours' notice of discharge was criticized by those who felt that he should be free to walk out at any given moment. Lord Russell admitted that 'in a purely legal and technical sense' this three days' restraint on a patient who wished to leave might be considered detention; but in fact it was a mere breathing-space—an opportunity for the patient to change his mind, for the hospital to make the necessary arrangements for his discharge, and to ascertain that he was not in a certifiable condition which would make him a danger to himself or to others.

Lord Dawson of Penn, who was perhaps the most eminent physician of his day, made an interesting plea for the development of community services from a medical point of view:

'The fact is that disease, if I may use the expression, breeds less and less true. It conforms less and less to type. In the days of acute infection ... the force of the external agent was such that it reduced the sufferers almost down to a common type, with the result that the type

[1] The second reading of the Bill, November 28th, 1929.

of illness was relatively easy and uncomplicated to treat and manage. But in these days, when the external agents are less strong, the colour and pattern of disease is more likely to be determined in greater degree by a man's make-up, his family history, his environment, the strain he has been liable to meet. The result is that you get a more complex picture than in days gone by.'

In the Commons, the Bill was introduced by the Rt. Hon. Arthur Greenwood, then Minister of Health, on December 23rd, 1929. He made it clear that the Bill embodied only 'the less controversial proposals of the Report'. No attempt had been made to abolish the 1890 Act. The intention of this Bill was to by-pass it—to provide a framework of treatment which would make it unnecessary to use the older Act, except in extreme cases.

Greenwood quoted extensively from the Macmillan Report of 1926, laying particular stress on its recommendations with regard to preventive work and early treatment. He pointed out the passing of the Local Government Act had facilitated the changes proposed.

A full House listened to the Minister. The debate which followed his speech went on until 4.0 a.m. During this time, the Board of Control came under considerable fire, and there were many speakers who thought that it would be an advantage if all its functions were to be transferred to the Minister direct. 'The mysterious and awful Board of Control,' Dr. Ethel Bentham[1] called it. 'People do not know of its name, or how to get at it.' 'An unapproachable body,' supplemented Jack Jones, M.P. for Rhondda, perhaps better known as the author of *Rhondda Roundabout*. 'You can write them letters, you can send appeals, but you get the same old stereotyped reply every time.' Dr. Bentham believed that there were still mistakes in certification, and that the public should not be lulled by the introduction of the 'voluntary' system into thinking that all was well. She instanced the case of a man who was found wandering, and was said to be suffering from mutism. He appeared silent and morose, refusing to answer any questions, or to give any account of himself, On an irrational impulse, Dr. Bentham spoke to him in French—and discovered that he was a Frenchman who spoke no English.

There was little serious criticism, apart from that directed at the Board of Control. Captain D. W. Gunston[2] called the Report 'one of

---

[1] Labour Member of Parliament for East Islington. Member of the Metropolitan Asylums Board.

[2] M.P. (Cons.) for Thornbury, Glos. and Parliamentary Private Secretary to the Minister of Health (Kingsley Wood) 1926–9. Now Major-General Sir Derrick Gunston.

the most magnificent reports which has ever been written' and spoke with some wonder of the lack of opposition to the main clauses of the Bill. 'We know,' he added, 'that, as a general rule, one only has to mention the liberty of the subject, and lawyers flock to the House, a sort of Habeas Corpus look comes over their faces. . . .' Possibly the 'Habeas Corpus look' was forestalled on this occasion by the fact that Lord Macmillan, Lord Jowitt and Lord Russell had already supported the Bill in the Lords.

Colonel Wedgwood, who had opposed the Mental Deficiency legislation of 1913 and 1927,[1] was absent from the first and second readings; but at the third reading,[2] he put down twenty questions, and spent some time recounting to the House the plot of G. K. Chesterton's novel *The Ball and the Cross*, in which more and more people are found to be insane until only a psychiatrist is left—and he reveals himself as the Devil. Eventually Col. Wedgwood suffered a rebuke from the patient Speaker: 'If the Rt. Hon. and gallant gentleman would only read the Bill. . . .'

Mr. W. J. Brown then took up the entertainment of the House by recounting the case of his sister, who had suffered from the delusion that she was being poisoned. A mental hospital wanted to practise forcible feeding. A Harley Street psychiatrist diagnosed dementia praecox, and said that the prognosis was hopeless. An elderly aunt of Mr. Brown's then gave the patient several doses of Epsom Salts, and she recovered in a few days.

The ramifications of this fascinating case might be discussed by psychiatrists for a very long time; but as far as the House was concerned, it was a mere debating point. Most of the discussion was serious and responsible, concerned with the detailed working of a new system which nearly all were agreed was desirable. Again the debate went on until the early hours of the morning. It was to be many years before the House again showed much interest in the mentally ill.[3] 'A very excellent Bill,' one member called it, 'and . . . a great charter for the poor of this country.' It received the Royal Assent on July 10th, 1930.

[1] See pp. 63-4 and 79.
[2] *Hansard*, April 11th, 1930.
[3] The next full-dress debate on mental health took place on February 19th, 1954.

Chapter Eight

THE MENTAL TREATMENT ACT, 1930

THE Mental Treatment Act did four things: it reorganized the Board of Control; it made provisions for voluntary treatment; it gave an official blessing to the establishment of psychiatric out-patient clinics and observation wards; and, in line with the Local Government Act of 1929, it abolished out-moded terminology, and brought the official expressions used in connection with mental illness more into line with the modern approach to the subject.

The Central Authority (sections 11–15)

The reorganization of the Board of Control provided for the establishment of a chairman and not more than five members, who were to be styled Senior Commissioners, and all of whom were to be salaried officials. One was to be a legal Commissioner, two were to be medical Commissioners, and one was to be a woman. There was no requirement that the woman member should possess either legal or medical qualifications.[1] The Senior Commissioners were to be appointed by the Crown on the recommendation of the Minister of Health, or of the Lord Chancellor in the case of the legal Commissioner.

The Senior Commissioners were to constitute the Board of Control. Their main task was to handle administrative work in London, and to supervise the visitation carried out by the other Commissioners. The visiting, or junior, Commissioners were to be appointed by the Board with the approval of the Minister of Health, and were, from the date of the appointed day under this Act, to be exclusively full-time and

[1] Of the four women Senior Commissioners serving 1930–59, three (Miss Dendy, Mrs. Pinsent and Miss Darwin) were lay and one (Dr. Wilson) medical.

salaried officials. Under the Mental Deficiency Act of 1913, unpaid Commissioners had been appointed; but the nature of the work was now so exacting that it was no longer a suitable sphere for voluntary public service.

The Local Authorities (sections 6–10 and 19)

County and county borough councils were authorized to make provision for the establishment of psychiatric out-patient clinics at general hospitals or mental hospitals, to make arrangements for after-care, and, with the consent of the Board of Control, to foster research[1] (section 6 (2)). Under section 19, patients liable to be detained in a workhouse under section 11 of the Lunacy Act 1890 could be sent instead to 'any . . . hospital or part of a hospital provided by the council of a county. . . .'[2]

Voluntary and Temporary Patients (sections 1–5)

The Macmillan Report had considered only two categories of patients—'Voluntary' and 'Involuntary'. The Act established three—'Voluntary', 'Temporary' and 'Certified'. The procedure for certified patients was already established under the Lunacy Act of 1890.

The procedure for voluntary patients was as follows: any person wishing of his own free will to undergo mental treatment (the Act used the phrase 'desirous of voluntarily submitting himself to treatment' which was perhaps unfortunate) could make a written application to the person in charge of any establishment approved by the Board of Control, and could be received as a patient without the necessity for a reception order.

In the case of a patient under sixteen, the volition was that of the parent or guardian, who could make a similar application, accompanied by a medical recommendation from a practitioner approved for this purpose by the Minister of Health or the local authority.

A voluntary patient might discharge himself at any time on seventy-two hours' notice. The essential nature of voluntary status involved the capacity of the patient to make a decision about his own treatment. If at any time he became incapable of such volition, he was to lose his

---

[1] These clauses gave the local authorities wide scope for action. Very few seem to have taken full advantage of them.

[2] Thus bringing mental treatment legislation into line with the intentions of the Local Government Act, 1929 (19 Geo. V, c. 17).

voluntary status. It would then be necessary to discharge him from hospital, certify him, or treat him as a temporary patient.

Temporary patients (section 5) were defined as persons 'suffering from mental illness and likely to benefit by temporary treatment, but for the time being incapable of expressing (themselves) as willing or unwilling to receive such treatment'. The intention was to provide for those cases where mental illness might be ascribed to a definite organic cause, such as childbirth or alcoholism, and where a relief of the physical condition might be expected to produce an improvement in the mental condition in a short space of time. Recognition as a temporary patient involved a petition from a near relative, and two medical certificates made out within five days of each other, and not more than fourteen days before reception into hospital.

If the patient regained the power of volition, he would be obliged either to make application for treatment as a voluntary patient, or to be discharged within twenty-eight days. The initial duration of a Temporary order was six months; this might be extended for two further periods of three months each with the permission of the Board of Control, but could in no case exceed one year in all.

Change of Terminology

The Local Government Act of 1929 had already swept away such terms as 'pauper' and 'Poor Law'. Now came the abolition of those outdated words which were still used officially in connection with mental illness. 'Asylum' was replaced by 'mental hospital' or simply 'hospital'; and 'lunatic'—except in certain specific legal contexts, such as 'criminal lunatic'—was replaced by a variety of phrases such as 'patient' or 'person of unsound mind' as the context might require. A 'pauper lunatic' was thus, by virtue of two Acts of Parliament, now a 'rate-aided person of unsound mind'.

Reactions to the Mental Treatment Act

In July, 1930—only a few days after the Act became law—the Board of Control held a two-day conference at the Central Hall, Westminster. It was attended by medical superintendents of county and county borough mental hospitals, by members of the Visiting Committees of such hospitals, by representatives of local health authorities, and by voluntary workers.

The general atmosphere was one of jubilation. The Act was hailed as being a long-overdue reform, and one which would in a short space of time revolutionize the treatment of the mentally ill. The work of the best authorities had been officially endorsed. The work of the less progressive authorities would now have to be brought up to standard.

An address was given by the Minister of Health, the Rt. Hon. Arthur Greenwood, in which he said:

'If this Act means anything at all, it means that we have ceased to think of mental disease as something that is so indecent that it has to be kept in a separate category of its own. . . . It has taken ten years and a Royal Commission to get where are today, and it has not been easy. . . . You asked for these powers: you have got them. I hope you will use them.'

There was no lack of goodwill to carry out the Minister's behest; but some speakers were already becoming aware of the difficulties inherent in the Act. It was an opportunity—but it was not a panacea. The real problems remained to be worked out in terms of administrative and medical practice.

Dr. Beaton, of the City Mental Hospital, Portsmouth, referred to a danger which was inherent in the creation of voluntary status: that the voluntary patients would form a kind of élite, receiving a better type of treatment and a greater proportion of available resources, than the certified patients. He stressed something which was already in danger of being overlooked—that voluntary and certified patients were not patients of differing social levels, persons of differing types of behaviour, or people suffering from different forms of illness. The sole difference between the two categories was that one had the power of volition, and wished to undergo treatment; the other either had not the power of volition, or resisted the suggestion of entering a mental hospital.

There was another problem also: that voluntary patients, being able to come and go almost at will, might consume a great deal of time and money without being cured or improved. They might enter hospital, and then refuse treatment. They might start on a course of treatment, and then leave without completing it.

A third problem, discussed by a number of speakers, was that of inducing patients to accept this new form of admission. The stigma of certification, of treatment as a 'pauper lunatic', was still very strong, and it would be many years before the old words and the old attitudes were finally eradicated.

The difficulties of getting voluntary patients into hospital; of seeing that they received full treatment where possible; of ensuring that certified patients did not suffer by comparison: all these were inherent in the Act; but to them was added another special difficulty, arising from the economic state of the country at that time. Between 1929 and 1931, the numbers of the unemployed more than doubled.[1]

As the numbers of the unemployed rose, unemployment benefit was repeatedly cut, and there were many people living lives of unwanted idleness near the starvation level. A hint of this social tragedy can be seen in a speech from Sir William Lobjoit:

'There are many people ... who would like to make a home in a mental hospital as a voluntary boarder. It would be a relief from standing from day to day outside an Employment Bureau, to have a home in one of the comfortable well-staffed mental hospitals we know of. We shall therefore have to be on our guard against the malingerers.'

Possibly some speakers felt that Sir William's view of existing mental hospitals, like his view of the popular attitude to mental illness, was over-optimistic; but the fact remains that, during this period, some mental hospitals did have difficulty in distinguishing those who were in real need of mental treatment from those whose primary need was a bed and four square meals a day. The danger of confusing the poor and the mentally sick had arisen again, this time in a different context.

Sir William's reference to 'well-staffed' mental hospitals needs perhaps a word of explanation, since only two or three years previously, there had been an acute staff shortage; but the very factor which had increased the number of would-be patients knocking at the doors of the mental hospitals had also increased the staff available. Other kinds of employment were hard to find; and there was, during these years of financial crisis, a considerable influx of new recruits, particularly men, into mental nursing. Many of them came from depressed areas—among them, small tradesmen, miners, and craftsmen. The hospitals usually required that they should be physically fit, and able either to take part in organized games or to play a musical instrument. On these slender qualifications, they started training; and although some went back into other employment when the crisis years were passed, a surprising number remained to make excellent trained mental nurses. Already, in 1930, we were learning that it is almost impossible to staff

[1] Ministry of Labour; Abstract of Labour Statistics. Percentage of insured persons unemployed; 1929-10·2; 1930-17·4; 1931-20·8.

mental hospitals in times of national prosperity; and only too easy in times of depression.

Temporary status was seen by most of the speakers at this Conference as a kind of half-way house between voluntary status snd certification. It was intended to involve no stigma; and it involved no judicial intervention. At the same time, it made provision for the treatment of non-volitional patients. The inherent difficulty here was in defining 'recovery of volition'. A patient might say, 'I want to go home' long before he was fit to make a settled judgment about his own future. He might demand his discharge one day, and be afraid to leave the hospital the next. There was no kind of precedent, medical, legal, or psychiatric for judging the existence of reasonable powers of volition on this point.

Out-patient clinics were more generally hailed as a settled and workable device. There seemed to be no difficulties here. 'All you need,' declared one speaker jubilantly, 'is a chair and yourself and a patient.' Dr. Good, of the Oxford County and City Mental Hospital, who was associated with an out-patient clinic started originally in 1916 to deal with shell-shock cases, thought that the general establishment of such clinics would inevitably lead in time to an increase in the right sort of voluntary patients. Patients who fought shy of mental treatment in the first place would go to a general hospital 'because they are not afraid of being locked up there or specially labelled. . . . A patient will not come to me, perhaps, as Dr. Good, the specialist of Littlemore, but he will come to me at the Radcliffe; and when I have treated him at the general hospital, he will then not care two straws whether he goes to see me at the Radcliffe or the mental hospital.'

He felt that another beneficial effect of the foundation of psychiatric clinics at general hospitals was that they generated among medical students a new and often intense interest in psychological medicine. From all aspects, the increasing links between general and mental hospitals were advantageous to both.

A further subject which received much attention at this Conference was that of after-care, and the relation of social work in mental illness to that of the general social services. The published report of the Conference contained an appendix describing the newly-inaugurated course for psychiatric social workers at the London School of Economics, and there is no doubt that this new development, financed by the Commonwealth Fund of America, was very much in the minds of those present. All agreed that social care was a necessary part of the patient's treatment and rehabilitation to conditions of normal living. Some contended, with Dr. Lord, that after-care was 'a definite part of clinical psychiatry—no longer a purely human and benevolent activity'; others felt that the task of integrating the patient back into normal society was one for the general social worker, who was in close touch with the other statutory services. Miss (later Dame) Evelyn Fox, who was then secretary of the Central Association for Mental Welfare, made a clear-cut and valuable statement on the task of a social worker. She also emphasized that any person undertaking this work should be trained. Social work was more than sympathy and common-sense. It was a skill which could be communicated, a technique to be acquired. Where a social worker worked in conjunction with a psychiatrist, her task was to provide him with the social background of the case, and then to act as his instrument in adjusting domestic situations where necessary. In the after-care phase, when the patient no longer needed psychiatric treatment, the social worker continued this difficult and delicate task of social readjustment until the patient was capable of managing his own situations.

The Conference was a great success. It ventilated a few grievances, raised a few doubts, and aired a few prejudices; but it was at the same time a most valuable instrument of discussion and of the propagation of new ideas. This was not the first Conference of this sort organized by the Board of Control; but the pattern was now set for many future fruitful meetings, in which all the parties concerned in operating mental health legislation might consider their joint problems.

DEVELOPMENTS 1930–9

The Report of the Board of Control for 1930 showed great satisfaction with the achievements of the new Act. It stressed that most of its provisions were permissive, and that 'it might be described in the main as an enabling measure'. The Conference which followed had been organized with the intention of encouraging the local authorities to use the Act to the fullest extent.

Accommodation for Voluntary and Temporary Patients

Although the Act had resulted in an immediate and startling increase in the number of out-patient clinics, little progress had been made in the task of setting aside special accommodation for the new categories of patients. This was partly a matter of cost. Lay committees were ready enough to agree to setting up psychiatric out-patient clinics, which required little capital expenditure, and represented an obvious saving of hospitalization costs. A new unit for voluntary patients, on the other hand, was a heavy charge on capital funds; and it was by no means easy to prove that the ultimate result of building such a unit would be to save money, because the patients would get better more quickly.

Another reason for this slowness of development was that many psychiatrists, like Dr. Beaton of Portsmouth, were not convinced as to the necessity for, or advisability of, special units. While they were agreed that beds should certainly be provided for voluntary patients, and that they should have the best treatment available, they felt that special accommodation would improve treatment for these patients at the expense of the certified patients. The stigma of certification would be increased; and there would be a tendency for the new units to be developed as 'show places' at the expense of the rest of the hospital.

Development of the use of voluntary procedure for admission was at first distinctly unequal. By the end of 1931, one area[1] could boast that 45 per cent of all admissions were voluntary; yet another, containing a total population of over four million people, had not admitted one voluntary patient by the summer of 1932.[2] In the subsequent years, however, voluntary admissions rose steadily. In 1932, the overall figure was 7 per cent of total admissions. By 1936, it was 26·9 per cent; and by 1938, it had risen to 35·2 per cent, while fifteen hospitals were admitting more than half their new patients in this way.

Conditions in Mental Hospitals

The re-constituted Board of Control was waging a vigorous battle for better conditions for all mental hospital patients. Annual Reports in the nineteen-thirties show a capacity for independent assessment, lively comment, and occasionally stinging rebuke. A note on the necessity for the provision of mental hospital libraries runs:

'Because patients are allowed to read anything, it must not be assumed that they will be content with any rubbish produced by past

[1] Un-named in the Board of Control's Annual Report, 1931.
[2] The Lancashire Mental Hospitals Board area. As a result of this comment by the Board of Control, 5 per cent of all beds in the area were made available for voluntary patients in the next year.

piety or present ineptitude. . . . A generation accustomed to Edgar Wallace will not, even in dementia, take kindly to Victorian sentimentality, or the "life and remains" of eminent divines.'

They suggested that the Red Cross of the local county library might supply suitable books, and added that clubs and hotels could often be induced to donate magazines.

Women patients had a champion—probably Dame Ellen Pinsent, who was now the woman Senior Commissioner of the Board. 'Only advanced dementia,' runs the 1932 Report, 'would reconcile the average woman to the type of garment still worn in some hospitals.' Two years later came the comment, 'A good hair cut and shampoo have a real tonic value . . . the woman who is content to wear her hair untrimmed and a frock like a sack certainly is not normal.' This recognition of the therapeutic value of clothes and hairdressing facilities was new to many hospitals, where committees were apt to consider such things as unjustifiable luxuries.

Food was important, too—and not merely as a means of existence. Patients needed to be reassured by familiar dishes ('a generation accustomed to fish and chips cannot be expected to eat steamed cod with anything but reluctance') and occasionally surprised by some special meal. This was not mere sentimentality on the Board's part. Many patients who came into mental hospitals in the period of economic depression were suffering from malnutrition; and more recent anthropological studies have shown that diet and the choice of food may be closely linked with mental health. Primitive communities have been found to deteriorate both mentally and physically when their own traditional dishes are replaced by the diet sheets of nutrition experts; and many a mental patient's re-socialization has begun under the influence of a good Christmas dinner.

In 1934, the Board of Control undertook a survey of entertainments and recreations provided in mental hospitals. They found that almost all hospitals had a programme of activities covering the whole year. There were frequent cinema shows, and sports such as cricket, football and hockey. A number of hospitals had organized dancing-classes. Most had regular dances for men and women patients, and were beginning to break down the rigid segregation of the sexes which had previously been the rule in mental hospital life. Segregation had been emphasized by the administrative pattern of mental hospitals, where the 'male side', headed by the chief male nurse, and staffed by male nurses, was separate from the 'female side', headed by the matron and staffed by female nurses.

The question of open and closed wards figures prominently in the Board of Control's reports at this time. The general practice was for almost all wards (the 'ward' comprising both day and night rooms for its patients) to be kept locked. Nursing and medical staff were accustomed to walk the hospital to the accompaniment of jangling bunches of keys, and for a nurse to lose his or her keys was the swiftest road to dismissal. Mental hospitals had long been dominated by the symbol of the locked door. Now the admission of voluntary patients indicated that more doors should be opened, and some patients at least should be free to come and go independently. The introduction of open wards at first aroused many tensions, particularly among the older nurses, some of whom found it difficult to adapt to the new situation; but it was found that, except where very disturbed patients were concerned, opening the doors was often a tranquillizing influence. The patient no longer felt that he was being 'locked away', and became more amenable as a result.

With the gradual introduction of the open door came the development of a parole system. Many patients could be given a limited degree of freedom, and be trusted to keep it. There developed a system of gradually extending parole as the patient's condition warranted it—'hospital parole', which meant that he could go anywhere in the building not specially out of bounds; 'ground parole', which enabled him to go as far as the outside gates of the hospital; and 'outside parole', which allowed him to go out alone, or with another patient, to visit relatives or to go into the nearest town at week-ends. Finally came 'week-end parole'—the patient being allowed home on trial for a short period before final discharge. The parole system has done much to break down the barriers between the mental patient and the community outside. The Board stressed year after year the importance of this system, and looked for its extension in all mental hospitals.

Professional Training

Training courses in psychiatry were now well organized. The Diploma in Psychological Medicine was offered by the Universities of London and Manchester, and the conjoint boards of England and Ireland. This was, and still is, the recognized post-graduate qualification for medical practitioners, and involved in most cases a two-year course, undertaken as a supplement to clinical work in a mental hospital. For a time, a short refresher course on a lower professional standard was organized at the Maudsley Hospital; and the University of London Extension Movement, in association with the Royal Medico-Psychological Association, arranged a yearly course of its own.

The Tavistock Clinic, founded in 1920, organized specialized courses on psycho-analytic lines, and stimulated research into the aetiology of neurosis.

Training for both male and female nurses was still organized by both the General Nursing Council and the R.M.P.A. The G.N.C. course took three years in an approved training school, or four years in an affiliated school. A State Registered Nurse could take the Mental Nursing Certificate in two or three years respectively. The R.M.P.A. course still operated separately, and was less exacting as far as theoretical knowledge—in allied subjects such as anatomy and physiology—was concerned.

Several universities now ran basic training courses for social workers. These courses, first founded in the Universities of London, Liverpool and Birmingham in the early years of this century, combined an academic course in social theory and social policy with practical work experience under supervision. By 1918, Miss Elizabeth Macadam, who had been responsible for the institution of the Liverpool course, had organized a national body—the Joint Universities Council for Social Studies—which made requirements with regard to professional qualifications. The universities gradually recognized these qualifications by the award of certificates and diplomas. The first degree course for social workers was instituted in the University of Manchester in 1937. Many avenues of social work were open to these workers, and a number found their way into the mental health field, practising social case-work in mental hospitals and out-patient clinics.

The specialized course in psychiatric social work[1] was at this time available only at the London School of Economics. The course lasted one year, and was open only to mature and experienced social workers, usually of some academic standing.

The first trained occupational therapist to work in England was Mrs. Glyn Owens, who trained in America, and set up a training school for occupational therapists in conjunction with Dr. Elizabeth Casson at Dorset House, Bristol, in 1930. The Association of Occupational Therapists was founded in 1936, and a system of qualifying examinations was started in 1938.

[1] See p. 124.

New Mental Hospitals

Two mental hospitals of the present day express the concept of mental treatment which was developed in the nineteen-thirties—Bethlem and Runwell. Bethlem was a charitable foundation with a very long and chequered history. Founded as a priory of the Order of St. Mary of Bethlehem in 1247, it received mental patients from 1377, and was for several centuries the only public hospital in England devoted to their care. In the eighteenth and early nineteenth centuries, Bethlem fell upon bad times. There were frequent allegations of corruption and maladministration, of poor treatment and neglect. After 1853, however, when the hospital was brought under the supervision of the Lunacy Commissioners, conditions improved considerably; and by 1930, Bethlem was again one of the foremost centres for the treatment of mental illness.

The hospital had already moved twice. The first Bethlem, in Bishopsgate, was left for a site in Moorfields in 1676. This second hospital was the 'Bedlam' of the eighteenth century. The third, at Southwark, was occupied in 1815. The fourth Bethlem is the present-day one, at Beckenham, in Kent. When the Southwark premises became overcrowded, and the limited space available too small for modern methods of treatment and occupation, the Court of Governors issued an appeal, and £50,000 was subscribed for a new building. This, completed in 1930, consists of a number of buildings, set in a park of 200 acres of land. Four houses were built for the patients, each with between 40 and 100 beds; and a nurses' home, a block of flats for married male nurses, and extensive science and treatment laboratories were constructed.

Bethlem remained a charitable foundation until 1948, though the patients it has received in this century have differed considerably from the 'Bedlam beggars' of earlier times. As the county asylums absorbed the insane poor, Bethlem drew its patients increasingly from the professional and middle classes. Many of these were people in straitened financial circumstances; but when the move to Beckenham took place in 1930, a proportion of patients were paying the full cost of maintenance.

Runwell was a completely new hospital—the first to be planned since the First World War, designed to embody new ideas in mental treatment. Larger than Bethlem, it had at the time of opening in 1937 a patient-population of 1,010; but this total was broken down into small units, each largely self-contained. Runwell is the only English mental hospital to be built entirely on the villa-system. Small one- or two-storey blocks with flat roofs were scattered over a wide area of garden and parkland. Parole patients, who required relatively little super-vision, were housed in units for twenty to twenty-five persons, where they might live something approaching a normal life, unhampered by the weight of institutionalism. Separate blocks were constructed for patients' clubs, where resocialization through group methods could be tried out; and a research wing was built and equipped for the examina-tion of the biochemical and neurological bases of mental disorder.

In both Bethlem and Runwell, the main emphasis in design and planning were the same: the breaking-up of the total patient popula-tion into smaller social groups; the provision of extensive grounds, to enable parole patients to have relative freedom of movement; the modern architectural design, unlike the Victorian barrack-pattern; the building and equipping of research laboratories. The appearance of these two hospitals differs from that of the late nineteenth-century mental hospitals as greatly as the 1930 Act differs from the Act of 1890 —and for the same reasons.

PART FOUR
Towards a Mental Health Service

Chapter Nine

FIRST STEPS IN INTEGRATION

DEVELOPMENT of the mental health services so far had been both divided and sporadic. The dichotomy between the services for the mentally ill and the mentally defective was complete. Some local authorities had developed services for one group, but had neglected the other. Some had neglected both. Where medical, nursing and social work staff were well qualified and enthusiastic, an excellent and efficient service had developed; but where the old ideas about mental deficiency and mental illness were still current, there was apathy and indifference. There was no effective central authority—for while the Board of Control was doing good work in bringing mental hospitals and mental deficiency institutions into line with modern social and psychiatric theory, those institutions no longer represented the whole range of available treatment. The community services—out-patient clinics, domiciliary visits by social workers, occupation centres, industrial centres, were of increasing importance; and though the Ministry of Health exercised a certain control over these activities of local health authorities, it was largely a financial control. The Ministry appears to have taken little positive action to encourage the development of more specialized services. The initiative lay with the energetic local authorities; the apathetic were allowed to rest in peace.

THE OXFORD MENTAL HEALTH SERVICES, 1937

Dame Ellen Pinsent was asked in 1937 if she would undertake a survey of the Oxford mental health services on behalf of the Oxford Delegacy for Social Studies. Dame Ellen was now a Senior Commissioner of the Board of Control, with a record of over thirty years' continuous association with the problems of mental disorder. Her report gives an interesting picture of the better type of provision available at that time.

Dame Ellen did not claim that the services she described were 'typical' of anything at all. Oxford, by reason of its traditions and its unusual population-structure, was very much of a special case; but she extended her survey over the counties of Oxfordshire and Berkshire, and was able to draw some illuminating comparisons with the city service.

The city of Oxford's mental health scheme was said to be the finest in England for diagnosis and early treatment. It was based on a belief in the paramount importance of maternity and infant welfare clinics, where abnormalities could be detected at the earliest possible stage. There were twelve such centres in the city. The City Council was responsible for the salaries of doctors and nurses, and for the rent of two centres. All other expenses were met from funds voluntarily subscribed. All mental health problems, whether in the mother or the child, were referred to the mental health services as a matter of routine.

There was a child guidance clinic, run by a team consisting of a general practitioner, a psychiatrist, and a social welfare worker. An observation school for problem children had been opened in 1930, where the reaction of these children to work and play situations could be studied over an extended period. There were 48 children, all suffering from personality disorders. The I.Q.s ranged from 70 to 95. Dame Ellen stressed that there was no organized after-care from this school, though the headmaster did a good deal of informal follow-up work on a personal basis. For retarded children, there were the usual 'special classes', operating in conjunction with the primary schools. Eight such classes dealt with 175 children. The special class children were not visited regularly by either a psychiatrist or an educational psychologist, and the child's progress was thus judged only by the teacher. Supervision of mental defectives in the city area was carried out by the Mental Welfare Association.

For adult patients, there were several types of provision—a county mental hospital, a registered hospital, an out-patient clinic, a colony for mental defectives, and, of course, the residuary services of Public Assistance. The County Mental Hospital, Littlemore, had 880 beds, no overcrowding, and no waiting-lists. The buildings were old, having been completed in 1846, but in good repair. The staffing position was good—a ratio of approximately one nurse to five patients. All sisters and male charge nurses possessed either the R.M.P.A. or the G.N.C. qualification. The matron and several others were doubly trained—that is, they had the general nursing training leading to State Registration as well as a Mental Nursing Certificate. Nearly all the wards were open, and suitable patients were allowed out of the hospital on parole. The patients were occupied during the day, either on occupational therapy or on suitable light work in the hospital, and there were frequent entertainments, such as cinema shows and dances. The main difficulty was that the hospital was not free to concentrate on acute cases of mental illness, for which its services were best suited. There were many mild senile dements, and many mental defectives, for whom no other accommodation could be found.

The Warneford Hospital was a private non-profit-making hospital for 'the educated classes'. Treatment was provided in pleasant conditions at an average cost of £4 8s. od. per patient per week. Since the patients were self-maintained, they could not be employed on utility services—sweeping, cleaning, gardening, laundry work, and so on—as were the patients in Littlemore. Dame Ellen found that this was in fact a disadvantage, since occupation was an integral part of treatment, and it was difficult to find substitute occupations to fill the whole day. There was a certain amount of occupational therapy; but on the whole the patients were less occupied, less useful, and more inclined to brood about their own inadequacies than those in the County Hospital.

Boro' Court Colony for mental defectives had been opened in 1934. There were 45 male and 157 female patients, all adults. All the patients were employed on utility services, and there were adequate recreational facilities. Most of the patients were allowed home from time to time on holiday leave; and there was a small holiday home at Caversham for the benefit of those unable to rejoin their families.

The out-patient clinic at the Radcliffe Infirmary had been opened in 1918. Patients came to it readily, because it was situated in a general hospital. The services of the medical staff who came from Littlemore, were given voluntarily, and the local authority lent a mental health visitor for social work. At the time of Dame Ellen's visit, there were 234 patients on the books.

The Public Assistance services presented a less happy picture. There were many mental defectives and mentally disordered persons in the two Oxford Public Assistance institutions, in addition to numbers of confused and incoherent old people. No psychiatrist visited them, and often the mental health authorities had no knowledge of them.

In fact, even in this, probably the most advanced service in the country, there were two overall criticisms to be made: failure to secure diagnosis by a properly qualified person—a psychiatrist or an educational psychologist, as the case might be; and failure to make referrals to the proper authority. The first was due to lack of knowledge on the part of the authorities concerned—they often had no understanding of the necessity for accurate diagnosis. The second was frequently due to the difficulty in deciding who was the 'proper authority'. The committees involved in mental health work at the local authority level included the Mental Health Committee, the Mental Deficiency Committee, the Asylum (Mental Hospital) Visiting Committee, the Public Assistance Committee, the Education Committee, and the Finance Committee. It is easy to understand why adequate referrals were often not made.

In the rural areas of Oxfordshire and Berkshire, the overall picture was far less encouraging. The county authorities were dealing with large areas containing a scattered and sparse population. The population of rural Oxfordshire was so small that a penny rate would raise only £2,500. There were no special classes, no facilities for observation work on behavioural problems, no out-patient clinics. The county sometimes sent cases to the out-patient clinic at the Radcliffe, but made no financial contribution to the running of this clinic. No duties were delegated to a local Mental Welfare Association, and ascertainment and supervision were carried out on a much smaller scale by the health visitor—who, however high her standards and conscientious her work, had no special training or interest in mental health.

There was one small occupation centre, and mental defectives were sometimes sent to Boro' Court. There was not even a Mental Deficiency Committee.

Dame Ellen's general conclusion was that, though the gross cases of mental defect or disorder would receive institutional care in time, no attempt was being made to secure early diagnosis and treatment, and the community services were almost non-existent. In Berkshire, the position was very similar. Forty per cent of all known mental cases were in Public Assistance Institutions.

The distinction in treatment was thus not between the rich and the poor, as it had been before 1930; but between the urban and the rural. The latter were the under-privileged class.

Dame Ellen's general conclusions from this brief survey were twofold: first, that the local authorities were not making the best use of the services already available; and second, that they had no incentive to improve on them. The lack of interest in or understanding of mental health problems could reach all down the line—from the committees and the Medical Officer of Health who ignored the whole subject except when it was thrust upon them, to the health visitor who was inclined to resist a mental health component in her work on the grounds that a particular patient was 'not bad enough to be put away'.

The implications of this study reached out far beyond the boundaries of Oxfordshire and Berkshire. These were the problems of many local authorities all over England. Dame Ellen suggested three methods for the improvement of local authority mental health services:

1. The appointment of a Medical Officer of Mental Health, either co-existent with or immediately subordinate to the Medical Officer of Health. If appointed to the subordinate position, he should have direct access to the relevant committees of the local authority.
2. A joint user agreement to be made for the use of psychiatric facilities where the areas of two or more local authorities formed an obvious geographical or administrative whole.
3. Each area so formed to employ at least one fully-trained psychiatrist for local authority work, principally for prevention and diagnosis.

Over twenty years later, Dame Ellen's proposals seem counsels of perfection as far as many areas are concerned; but similar devices have been adopted in some of the more progressive and administratively homogeneous areas.

THE VOLUNTARY MENTAL HEALTH SERVICES: THE FEVERSHAM REPORT

In 1939, public interest switched from the work of local authorities to that of voluntary associations. These, as we have seen, had a long history in the field of community work, particularly in mental deficiency. They had grown up piece-meal, in response to special needs, as voluntary services often do; and the time had come when effective community work depended on co-ordination of effort.

This was the outstanding conclusion of the members of the Feversham Committee, which made its report to the Ministry of Health in 1939. The members of this Committee all had a long personal association with the problems involved. They included the Earl of Feversham, who was the current President of the Child Guidance Council; Sir

Henry Brackenbury, Vice-president of the British Medical Association, and also Vice-president of the Tavistock Clinic (see p. 129); Dame Katherine Furse, Director of the Women's Royal Naval Services; Lord Horder, the King's Physician; the Earl of Listowel, later Postmaster General, and then a Labour member of the London County Council; and Mrs. Montague Norman, (later Lady Norman), who was associated with the work of the Central Association for Mental Welfare and the Child Guidance Council.

The Report included a short account of the history of the mental health services, a review of existing conditions, and a series of recommendations for future action. The historical account is a little misleading, less because of its occasional inaccuracies of fact than because of the particular emphasis which the experience of the Committee's members tended to give it. The emphasis on community development, particularly through voluntary agencies, tends to detract from a full appreciation of the part played by the statutory authorities in reform and development.

In 1939, four voluntary associations operated on a national scale in the mental health field. These were the Mental After-Care Association, founded in 1879, which helped patients discharged from mental hospitals;[1] the Central Association for Mental Welfare, founded as the National Association for the Care of the Feeble-Minded in 1896, and reconstituted in 1913 to organize the community care of mental defectives under the new Act through its local associations; the National Council for Mental Hygiene, founded in 1918, which concentrated on educational and preventive work, and maintained links with similar organizations in other countries; and the Child Guidance Council, founded in 1927. There were also many local clinics, some operating in conjunction with local authorities, which appeared to be unattached to any central society.

Four separate associations had thus been created in response to four distinct needs. In some areas, their work overlapped, because the field of operation could not be neatly divided into four. In others, particularly in rural districts, there was no provision at all. Sometimes a single society was found to be carrying an overwhelming quantity of work for which its small staff and slender budget were wholly inadequate.

The first conclusion of the Committee was obvious: whatever the cost in personal loyalty, the four associations should amalgamate, to form a national Mental Health Association.

[1] See p. 105.

In a review of legislation for the mentally ill, the Feversham Committee deprecated the effects of the 1890 Lunacy Act, and stressed the need for full-scale revision of existing legislation to meet the new developments in the treatment of psychoneurosis. The 1930 Act had done much to improve the situation, but its implications had not yet been fully recognized throughout the country. Out-patient clinics were generally ill-equipped, under-staffed, and had inadequately trained personnel. The Committee considered that an adequate team in such a clinic would consist of a psychiatrist and a psychotherapist, both of whom should be on the staff of the local mental hospital, and employed on a sessional basis; a psychologist; a psychiatric social worker; and a secretary. It was clear that the theory of out-patient work had travelled a long way since, in 1930, Dr. Petrie had needed only a chair and himself and a patient.

The increase in voluntary admissions was encouraging. Temporary status, on the other hand, was being used very little. There was some uncertainty as to the type of case which was eligible; and the awkwardness and expense of procedure, together with the fact that the order had to be extended after six months if the patient had not recovered, meant that it was seldom employed.

In the mental deficiency services, shortages and inadequacies were everywhere to be seen. There was a great lack of occupation centres and special schools. There appeared to be no generally-accepted definition of what mental deficiency was, and the deciding factor in an individual case was too often the I.Q. which could be measured easily, rather than the degree of social adaptation, which could not.

The reason for this general failure of the mental health services was primarily the lack of public knowledge and interest in the work. Many local authorities, when asked if they carried out mental health education, replied that the subject was 'taboo', and that there was 'no demand' for such education. To the Feversham Committee, the fact that the subject was taboo was precisely the reason for starting educational work.

Some local authorities had pointed out that while general health education could be undertaken on a popular level by posters and slogans, such means were inappropriate for mental health propaganda. The Feversham Committee thought that more subtle approaches might be used.

Educational work had been sponsored with some success by a few mental hospitals, where the staff had set themselves the task of integrating the hospital with the local community. Lectures and informal talks had been given to a variety of local groups—Church organizations, youth clubs, and so on. A general letter to relatives, to be given to them on the patient's admission, could be framed to reassure them, and to give them some information about the hospital's work and the changing attitudes to mental illness. Some hospitals had instituted an occasional 'Open Day', when the general public could see the work for themselves. The dissemination of information could be a powerful force in overcoming the stigma which still remained.

On a different level, the work which the voluntary associations had undertaken with professional bodies, such as general practitioners and teachers, had a great value.

The Feversham Committee made many recommendations, ranging over a wide field. The most outstanding of these were as follows:

1. *Voluntary Societies:* Amalgamation of the four main central agencies—the Mental After-Care Association, the Central Association for Mental Welfare, the National Council for Mental Hygiene and the Child Guidance Council—to take place at the earliest practicable date.

2. *Educational Work:* The new national association to undertake the encouragement of educational work of all kinds, through local authority staff, mental hospital staff, and local voluntary associations.

3. *Mental Health Social Workers:* A minimum standard and a national qualification to be established, accompanied by a rise in status and salary-scale.

4. *Mental Hospital Services:* Out-patient clinics to be increased. Mental hospitals to work in close conjunction with the universities (for research purposes), the general hospitals (for border-line and 'observation' cases) and the local authorities (for community care).

5. *Mental Deficiency:* The criterion of 'social inefficiency' to be generally adopted. Special schools and occupation centres to be extended.

Many of the Feversham Committee's recommendations were in the nature of hopes for the future rather than concrete recommendations for immediate action. The amalgamation of three of the four voluntary associations was to take place under emergency conditions later in 1939; the integration of mental hospitals with medical schools and general hospitals was in some measure achieved by the National Health Service Act of 1946,[1] and the question of the training and status of mental health social workers has been taken up by the Mackintosh and Younghusband Committees.[2] The great value of this Report, apart from these factors, lay in its unhesitating emphasis on the community aspects of the Mental Health Services.

1939-45: THE SECOND WORLD WAR

The outbreak of war in September 1939 made the full implementation of the Report impracticable for the time being, and brought a crop of special problems. Inevitably, all the existing shortages were accentuated. As in the 1914-18 war, many doctors were called for service with the Forces. Some mental hospitals were taken over for emergency purposes—such as military or air-raid casualties, or to provide general hospital accommodation outside densely-populated areas—their patients being crowded into other hospitals, already full. Out-patient clinics collapsed for want of trained staff, or staff of any kind. Male nurses in the Territorial and Reserve Forces were called up. Some female nurses left to work in munitions. Those mental hospitals which continued their normal work faced all the problems of institutional life in war-time—acute shortages of clothing, food and heating—plus an unprecedented degree of overcrowding and understaffing. This meant the return of the locked door, of inactivity, of isolation.

At the same time, mental health work received a new and wider significance. The extension of the war to the civilian population meant that public morale was a major factor in victory or defeat.

There was a general fear in psychiatric circles in 1939 that the outbreak of war would be followed by widespread mental breakdown.[3] The whole community was in a state of extreme apprehension. Books such as Beverley Nichols's *Cry Havoc*, which forecast the end of civilization and an international holocaust if war were declared, had a wide circulation. Films such as 'The Gap', which depicted the effect of a major air-raid on an unprepared London in all its horror, were shown

[1] See p. 149.
[2] See pp. 159-60, 162-4.
[3] See R. Titmuss, *Problems of Social Policy*, p. 20, note.

to large and fearful audiences. By the time of Munich, public apprehension was so great that the issue of gas-masks, the erection of air-raid shelters, the digging of trenches in public parks and back gardens, the general acceptance of the inevitable, actually relieved the tension.

The administrative and medical problems consequent on public panic —and it seemed that such panic could easily be triggered off by the outbreak of hostilities—could be enormous. In October, 1938, a committee of psychiatrists from the London teaching hospitals was set up to consider the formation of a nation-wide mental health service to meet such a situation.

The Committee came to the conclusion that the conditions of war would so lower the threshold to stress that three to four million acute psychiatric cases could be expected within six months of the outbreak of war. To deal with these cases, an elaborate scheme involving local treatment centres, mobile psychiatric teams and special neurosis hospitals was suggested.

It is doubtful whether sufficient resources could have been spared under war conditions, or whether any resources would have been adequate to meet the problems envisaged. By the summer of 1940, it was clear that the Committee's estimate had, happily been wide of the mark. The effect of heavy bombing was to raise civilian morale rather than lowering it. The spirit of urban populations in England during the 'blitz' is something which has not yet been adequately explained; there was fear, but no panic; material destruction, but mental and spiritual survival.

Yet, if war did not produce the mass hysteria which had been feared, it certainly produced psychiatric problems of a varied nature. Among these were the problems consequent on evacuation. In Professor Titmuss's descriptive phrasing 'Every conceivable kind of psychological misfit, Conservative and Labour supporters, Roman Catholics and Presbyterians, lonely spinsters and loud-mouthed boisterous mothers, the rich and the poor, city-bred Jews and agricultural labourers, the lazy and the hard-working, the sensitive and the tough, were thrown into daily intimate contact'. The abrupt change of living conditions, the mixing of social and occupational classes, brought less dramatic problems than had been envisaged. There was no mass panic. Instead, undramatically, there was an increase in enuresis among children, and in psychosomatic disorders among adults.

To meet the new needs of war-time society, a Mental Health Emergency Committee had been set up by three of the four voluntary associations in 1939, following the recommendations of the Feversham Committee.[1] Three years later, this became the Provisional National Council for Mental Health. Its work in the provinces was based on the thirteen Civil Defence regions. It included supervision of evacuation problems, the rehabilitation of those unable to stand the strain of changed conditions, and a host of *ad hoc* activities which in retrospect are difficult to classify. By 1944, its workers were also dealing with the after-care of Service personnel discharged on psychiatric grounds. Each of the thirteen regions had an office, staffed by two or three workers, some of them psychiatric social workers, and others drawn from the societies which had amalgamated. The amount of work which could be done was strictly limited in scope by the small size of the organizations; but it was of great value in many individual cases, and formed a nucleus from which work in the provinces could later be developed.

THE MENTAL HEALTH SERVICES IN 1946

An important study which was to have considerable effect on the development of the post-war mental health services was Dr. C. P. Blacker's *Neurosis and the Mental Health Services*, published in 1946. This study was begun in 1942 on the suggestion of Dr. Aubrey Lewis, Clinical Director of the Maudsley Hospital, in order to survey the country's psychiatric resources in war-time. It was continued under the sponsorship of the Ministry of Health in order to make proposals for a new psychiatric service; and though Dr. Blacker's final recommendations were not official, they carried considerable weight in official circles.

The Report was primarily concerned with community services—which at that time meant only out-patient clinics; but it gave some interesting pointers for the future. (Incidentally, the title is an interesting example of that cleavage between the treatment of neurosis and the treatment of psychosis which the new National Health Service was to end.)

General practitioners on the whole retained a deep-seated prejudice against psychiatry. Blacker comments:

'The neurosis survey has shown that there exists throughout much of the country prejudices against psychiatry . . . there is in the provinces a

---

[1] The Mental After-Care Association remained a separate organization.

fairly widespread disinclination to utilize the psychiatric services which already exist . . . the main cause is a failure on the part of many general practitioners to appreciate the character of these services, an unawareness of the nature and prevalence of neuroses, and a widespread mistrust of psychiatry, largely focussed on analytic procedures, which are considered a decadent and modern fad.'

Blacker recommended that there should be closer links between general and mental hospitals, and that there should be better prospects for clinicians in mental hospitals. At that time, the only prospect of advancement was to the post of medical superintendent or deputy medical superintendent. This often meant that in a large hospital, a good clinician would be lost to clinical work and would have to apply himself to the unfamiliar and possibly uncongenial task of administration.

The total psychiatric services recommended by this survey were as follows: an increase of 75–100 per cent in out-patient clinics in the next five years; three or four mental hospitals of a maximum of 1,000 beds to one million people—the existing provision was roughly 3,000 beds to one million population, but these were largely in big hospitals with a thousand or more patients; at least one psychiatric social worker to each mental hospital—there were then 27 for 101 hospitals; a doubling of the existing institutional provision (46,000) for mental defectives; and a hundred beds per million population outside mental hospitals—that is, in teaching units or in general hospitals in large towns.

Existing provision when the Health Service came into operation was very much below the optimum framed by Dr. Blacker.

Chapter Ten

THE NATIONAL HEALTH SERVICE

W HILE the war was in progress, and even when its outcome seemed at times doubtful, plans for social reconstruction were being actively discussed. Among these was the plan for a national health service, including the mental health services.

The Beveridge Report on Social Insurance and the Allied Services, published in 1942, had made it clear that, if want in its grosser forms was to be abolished in England, three 'basic assumptions' must be made: the provision of children's allowances, a policy of full employment, and a national health service. From this basis came the series of interlocking pieces of legislation which in 1946-8 were to create the Welfare State.

A national health service was not only socially desirable, but also administratively inevitable. The piece-meal provision of the pre-war years, complex of voluntary hospitals, municipal hospitals and Public Assistance hospitals, had been hammered into a single service by the necessities of war. An emergency medical service, divided into twelve regions, each with a senior hospital officer, had already created a nation-wide hospital service on war footing. As early as 1940, a Medical Planning Commission consisting of representatives of the British Medical Association and the two Royal Colleges had been set up 'to study war-time developments, and their effects on the country's medical services, both present and future'.

The Beveridge proposals gave an added impetus to these movements, and put the whole question on a wider basis. Beveridge stressed that the development of a social insurance scheme which would provide adequate benefits in time of sickness was contingent on a reduction in the frequency and duration of sickness. A national health service 'should provide full preventive and curative treatment of every kind to every citizen without exceptions, without remuneration limit, and without an economic barrier at any point to delay recourse to it'.

In 1943, discussions between the Ministry of Health and the interested parties—in particular, the British Medical Association, representatives of the voluntary hospitals, and representatives of the local authorities—began. In April of that year, the Minister of Health stated in Parliament that the new scheme for a national health service would not include the mental health services;[1] but this decision was a short-lived one. The mental health services were included in the scheme set out by the White Paper of 1944, which quoted from the Report of the Macmillan Commission of 1924-6 in stressing that there was an interaction between mind and body, and that it was unreal to develop services for one without reference to the other.

A report, *The Future Organization of the Psychiatric Services* was published in June, 1945. This was a result of deliberations between representatives of the Royal Medico-Psychological Association, the Psychological Medicine Section of the B.M.A. and the Royal College of Physicians. The report stressed that 'the argument for treating psychiatry in all essential respects like other branches of medicine' was 'strong and conclusive . . . there is everything to be said for making the admintrative structure of psychiatry exactly the same in principle and even in major detail as that of other branches of the health services'.

The advantages of full integration were manifest. It would give the psychiatric services parity of esteem with other branches of medicine. It would end the artificial divorce between the treatment of the mind and the treatment of the body which had become impossible to maintain with the development of psychosomatic medicine. It would increase the available resources, end the cleavage between the treatment of psychoses (mainly carried out in county mental hospitals) and the neuroses (mainly carried out in large voluntary hospitals associated with the teaching of psychiatry, in out-patient clinics, or in private practice) and reduce the stigma which still attached to the mental patient.

The disadvantages of full integration were largely administrative. In the new Health Service, the local authorities were to be given wide powers in community care; but the hospitals were to be removed from the care of the local authorities, and placed under joint boards,[2] while

[1] *Hansard,* April 15th, 1943.
[2] The National Health Service Act substituted Regional Hospital Boards for the original proposal of joint boards for local authority areas.

general practitioners were to be dealt with by a third branch of the service, the Executive Councils. The patient would thus pass from the care of one branch to the other, and back again. He might begin by being under the care of his family doctor; go into a mental hospital for a time; be discharged to the care of the local authority mental health service; and finally return to the care of his family doctor again. Like many mental patients since 1930, he might return to the mental hospital for short periods of treatment from time to time. In all this, continuity of care could be lost, because the service was to operate in three sections which had little connection with one another.

Many people in the mental health field were aware of this difficulty. The problem was not entirely confined to the psychiatric services, since it affected two other fields where continuity of care before, during and after hospitalization was of special importance—the tuberculosis services and the maternity services. The proposal that these three services should remain in the hands of the local authorities was widely canvassed; but this could only be done at the sacrifice of total integration, the perpetuation of the idea that these services existed in isolation, apart from the general stream of medicine and public health work. The dilemma was absolute. In the circumstances, the decision to proceed with full integration, even at the cost of administrative trichotomy, was a wise one. It was widely endorsed by the medical profession in the columns of the *Lancet* and the *British Medical Journal*.

The National Health Service Act: Provisions relating to Mental Health

The main body of the Act contained few specific references to mental illness. The mental health services were to form part of the comprehensive health service for England and Wales. The former county mental hospitals, like other hospitals, were to come under the authority of the new Regional Hospital Boards.[1] Local authorities were charged with the 'prevention, care and after-care of illness and mental defectiveness'[2]—'illness' including both mental and physical illness.

The Minister of Health now became the central authority for mental health.[3] The Board of Control continued as an independent body, and retained its quasi-judicial interest in the liberty of the subject. Its Commissioners and Inspectors were still empowered to visit mental hospitals and mental deficiency institutions, to review individual cases, and

---

[1] Section 11 and schedule III.   [2] Section 28.   [3] Section 1.

to receive statutory documents relating to admission and discharge; but the Minister assumed responsibility for the administration of hospitals and institutions, the licensing of private homes and hospitals for the mentally disordered, and the control of local authority work.

The Central Health Services Council, which was to be the main advisory body, was to include among its forty-one members two medical practitioners and two laymen with knowledge and experience of the mental health services.[1] There was also to be a Standing Mental Health Advisory Committee, which might advise both the Minister and the Central Council.[2]

Local authorities acquired wide powers under section 28 of the Act in 'prevention, care and after-care'. The local Health Committee now took over the statutory duties previously carried out by the Public Assistance Committee and the Mental Deficiency Committee. Their full duties in relation to mental health were:

(a) The initial care and removal to hospital of persons dealt with under the Lunacy and Mental Treatment Acts.

(b) The ascertainment and (where necessary) removal to institutions of mental defectives, and the supervision, guardianship training and occupation of those in the community, under the Mental Deficiency Acts.

(c) The prevention, care and after-care of all types of patients, so far as this was not otherwise provided for.[3]

While the duties under the first two heads were statutory duties, the last section, covered in section 28 of the Act, was permissive. The actual phrase used shows some ambiguity:

'Local authorities may, and to such extent as the Minister may direct, shall . . . make provision. . . .'

There was thus a hint of possible future mandatory action, but a wide scope was in fact given to local authorities in their implementation of section (c).

The result was inevitably a great variation in practice. Some authorities rose to the challenge, notably in the large towns, and initiated a new mental health scheme which provided comprehensive care. Others were content to carry on with the statutory duties, without attempting

[1] Section 2 and schedule 1(i) e.
[2] Constituted under section 2 (iii).
[3] National Health Service Act 1946: Provisions relating to the Mental Health Services Published by the Ministry of Health and the Board of Control, 1948.

to do more than was mandatory upon them. Some set themselves to work to find means of co-operation and co-ordination with the hospital services, to ensure continuity of care. Others remained in comparative isolation.

In the mental hospitals, too, considerable changes took place as a result of the Act. The responsible authority was now the Regional Hospital Board, whose area centred on the university medical school.[1] This brought the practice and the teaching of psychiatry closer together, and enabled the mental hospitals, which generally existed in geographical and professional isolation, to form closer contacts with the teaching factilities of the Region. The only hospital group at first designated purely as a post-graduate teaching hospital for the psychiatric services was the Bethlem and Maudsley Group.[2]

Regional Hospital Boards were charged with the duty of setting up Hospital Management Committees, each of which would administer a small group of hospitals. No central direction was given as to whether mental hospitals should be grouped separately, or whether a single mental hospital might be included in general groups with hospitals of other types. Again there was a variation in practice: in one or two regions, notably Leeds and Birmingham, the latter policy was followed where geographical consideration made it advisable, though some mental hospitals were so large that they required a hospital management of their own. A typical group might contain a general hospital, a tuberculosis hospital, a maternity hospital, a mental hospital and a convalescent hospital—thus providing for all the varied needs of an area. This created some problems, since the traditional administration of a mental hospital is very different from that of other types of hospital.[3] In other regions, this difference of administration was considered so important that mental hospitals, even though some miles apart, were grouped together under Hospital Management Committees of their own. The dilemma at local level was precisely that which had been faced at the centre: was it better to safeguard the special needs of the mental patient at the risk of separating off the mental health services from other

[1] An interesting feature is the speed with which R.H.B. Areas were determined. A detailed draft of proposed areas was sent to interested bodies on November 15th, 1946, and the Determination of Regional Hospital Areas Order was laid before Parliament on December 18th, only four and a half weeks later. There was thus very little time for local consultation.

[2] A 'teaching hospital' is a hospital operating in close conjunction with a university medical faculty, and has a Board of Governors which is not responsible to the Regional Hospital Board. Other hospitals also have teaching facilities.

[3] See pp. 165–73.

branches of the Health Service, or to press ahead with full integration at the sacrifice of those special needs? Regional Boards varied in their answer to this question.

As far as the psychiatric services were concerned, it can be seen that the National Health Service Act provided for a firm central framework, but for considerable administrative flexibility at local level. In the early, experimental stages of the new service, this was all to the good. All though there were plenty of problems to be worked out in practice—and some of them are far from being solved yet—the basic structure allowed room for experiment and initiative. In doing so, it had inevitably to leave room for a certain amount of apathy, for false starts and doubtful decisions. This was the reverse side of the coin.

Nearly two years of questioning and preparation lay between the passing of the Act and the appointed day. On July 5th, 1948, as Sir James Stirling Ross says in a rare poetic moment, 'The whole gigantic scheme wheeled into line. It was like the slow opening of the immense hydraulic doors of the vaults of a great bank.'[1] Controversies had held up development, and recrimination was not yet finally stilled; but the scheme, ready or not, had to go forward, in order to synchronize with other major schemes of social change which formed the basis of the new Welfare State.

The National Health Service Act meant many things to many people: to general practitioners, a period of serious overwork; to former voluntary hospitals, frustration, and chafing under unfamiliar controls; to local authorities, new responsibilities and opportunities in an expanding field: to members of Regional Hospital Boards and Hospital Management Committees, new powers: to medical specialists, new possibilities of knowledge and professional advancement; but the most important single factor was its effect on the patient. By dissociating medical care and treatment from the ability to pay for it, by making free treatment available as of right and not as of charity, the Act brought freedom from fear for many who had never been able to afford adequate medical treatment, and who had suffered mental and physical disabilities from which they had no hope of recovery.

[1] J. S. Ross, *The National Health Service*, p. 128.

Chapter Eleven

PROBLEMS AND EXPERIMENTS, 1948-59

BETWEEN the appointed day of the National Health Service Act and the passing of the Mental Health Act is a period of a little over eleven years. As far as the mental health services are concerned, the two pieces of legislation are complementary. The period between them thus had an unusually transitional character.

Many of the developments referred to in this chapter are still in progress at the time of writing; and it is not easy to separate the inevitable teething troubles of a new service from permanent and intractable problems, or ephemeral fashions in thought and practice from long-term progress. Future assessment of these eleven complex years may find trends where at present there is only confusion and contradiction, points of emphasis which a contemporary survey overlooks. This chapter represents only an interim assessment.

The great change since 1948 has been the entry of statutory authorities into the field of community work, and the consequent change in the role of voluntary organizations. Local authority Mental Health Departments have begun to shoulder the burden of community care. Mental hospitals have taken up the theme of 'community' in two ways —by the development of a dynamic within the hospital which enables it to approximate more closely to the society from which its patients are drawn, and by the development of extramural psychiatric services which bridge the gap between total hospitalization and local authority care. Community services for mental defectives date back to the 1913 Act, which provided for supervision and guardianship, and occupation centres have a history of nearly forty years; but services for the mentally ill were originally conceived of in a more rigid way. Out-patient clinics were the first attempt to break away from the concept of the institution as the only means of treatment apart from charity or the Poor Law. Since 1948, local authority care, day and night hospitals, sheltered workshops and other experimental forms of care have done much to break down the old distinction between being totally well (at home) and totally sick (in hospital). We have begun to provide a flexible range of services to meet the varying needs of individuals.

The greatest barrier to the development of a full range of community services is the artificial division between local authority, general practitioner and hospital services introduced by the National Health Service Act. We have seen how this was the price which had to be paid for an integrated health service. The alternative—the exclusion of the mental health services from the general pattern of health provision in order to keep continuity of care—would have meant a great loss of status and of opportunities for progress. Integration was worth the price; but it has meant that a great deal of energy has had to be expended on liaison problems between the three branches of the service at local level.

These problems are acute. They are exacerbated by the fact that local authority boundaries and the boundaries of hospital catchment areas bear no relation to one another. In Lancashire, for example, there are within the Regional Hospital Board area seventeen county boroughs, each operating its own mental health service, and seventeen divisions of the County Council. One local authority may have patients in eight or nine different hospitals. One hospital may have patients from thirteen or fourteen different local authority areas. Liaison is tenuous, and difficult to maintain. An outstanding example is that of Barrow, which has to send patients to hospital in Lancaster, fifty miles away. It is often impossible for all the workers concerned with a single patient to get to know one another personally; sometimes the issue of confidentiality is raised between workers of different professional backgrounds. Mutual mistrust between general practitioners and psychiatrists, between medical practitioners as a whole and social workers, and between social workers of different backgrounds and training, means that written referrals are not always adequate, and sometimes do not exist at all.

The Central Health Services Council, in a report published in 1952,[1]

---

[1] Report on Co-operation between Local Authority, Hospital and Practitioner Services. S.O. No. 32-419, 1952.

pointed out that there were always severe administrative problems in large-scale organizations. The National Health Service had become the third largest concern in the country, employing over half a million people. Centralization involved one set of problems; devolution on a geographical or functional basis would have involved another. 'The greater the delegation to the periphery, the greater the problem of maintaining internal cohesion'. Either way, there were no easy answers.

The Report saw the problems of trichotomy as inevitable, but stressed that they had produced a serious situation in administrative practice. Co-ordination existed only at national level, in the Ministry of Health. Below that level, the three branches functioned separately; and even within each branch, there was no uniform and unitary structure. The hospital service contained both Regional Hospital Boards and independent Boards of Governors of teaching hospitals; the local authority service was complicated by local government boundaries, which separated county boroughs administratively from the surrounding county areas; and in the general practitioner services, local professional committees operated separately from Executive Councils. Over all was the problem of 'numbers and geography'. The Regional Hospital Board areas, based on university medical schools, bore no relation to local authority areas. One Regional Hospital Board area might contain a dozen or more local authorities and Executive Councils, whose areas also did not coincide with each other's. A reverse situation existed in the London area, where one local health authority (the L.C.C.) covered an area split between four Regional Hospital Boards, containing in all twenty-five Hospital Management Committees and twenty-six independent Boards of Governors. Rarely was it possible to work out a simple relationship between a Hospital Management Committee, an Executive Council, and a local health authority. 'The geographical pattern,' concluded the report, 'is so complicated that any one authority must find it difficult to be conscious of its opposite number.'

The report listed mental health, tuberculosis, maternity and child welfare and geriatric services as those in which it was most necessary to find ways of overcoming the disadvantages of tripartite structure. In all these services, there could be no clear-cut distinction between care and after-care, and continuity of service was all-important. In the mental health services in particular, 'systematic provision for co-operation' was 'imperative'.

Local authorities needed the expert psychiatric advice which only mental hospital staff could give them. Psychiatrists needed detailed information about their patients' home circumstances which could generally only be obtained from the local authority.[1] Both needed to combine on the task of following up discharged patients, and on the question of finding beds for new admissions. (This last question had become a point of friction in many regions; the local authorities were responsible for submitting cases for admission to mental hospitals and mental deficiency hospitals, but those hospitals necessarily determined priority of admission for themselves. In some areas, bed bureaux had been set up at regional level, to which local authority mental health workers could apply; but in others, the worker often had to contact several hospitals in succession; and between the worker's determination to find a bed for his patient and the hospital's determination to avoid further over-crowding, the situation often developed into a personal battle of wits.)

Existing methods to improve co-operation at local level included inter-locking membership between the different statutory authorities, the exchange of papers between authorities, *ad hoc* meetings at officer or committee level to exchange information or reach decisions, and *ad hoc* co-operation between individuals. Interlocking membership was provided for by the National Health Service Act, which had laid down that Regional Hospital Boards should include nominees of the university, the medical profession and the local health authorities in its area;[2] that Hospital Management Committes should include nominees from the local health authorities and the Executive Council;[3] that Boards of Governors of teaching hospitals should include nominees from the local health authorities and the Regional Hospital Board;[4] and that Executive Councils should have eight of their twenty-five members appointed by the local health authority.[5]

Ad hoc meetings and co-operation were perhaps the most valuable means of healing the existing divisions. 'If there were always close co-operation between officers, few difficulties would arise ... (but) one must look for other means which will work where personalities are conflicting or where officers ... overlook the effect of their actions upon others.' The Report concluded that joint health consultative committees should be set up for 'local health service areas'. These areas should

---

[1] Some mental hospitals had their own psychiatric social workers, who undertook domiciliary visiting.

[2] National Health Service Act, 1946, schedule 3, part I.

[3] Op. cit., schedule 3, part II.

[4] Op. cit., schedule 3, part III.

[5] Op. cit., schedule 5, part I.

be based on a County Borough or other large town, and the extent of the area should be determined by geographical and administrative considerations, by local agreement between the parties concerned. One or two Hospital Management Committees might thus find it convenient to meet members of the county borough health authority, the county health authority for the surrounding area, and the Executive Council or Councils which covered the same population.

LOCAL AUTHORITY SERVICES

Problems of Co-operation

In fact, very few local authorities have been able to use the device of the joint health consultative committee with any marked degree of success. As the Central Health Services Council had itself pointed out, the problems of 'numbers and geography' were intractable as far as present local authority boundaries were concerned.

The plan of centring an area service on a county borough is workable for other branches of the Health Service, since the hospitals for the area are probably within the county borough boundaries; but mental hospitals and mental deficiency institutions are seldom so placed. They were generally built in rural areas, away from centres of population. This was partly because country land is cheap, and mental hospitals require more land than general hospitals. A general hospital can build upwards, and does not need extensive grounds, while a mental hospital, with a largely ambulant population, has to be constructed to give the patients access to walks and gardens; and open-air activities have traditionally formed part of mental hospital programmes. Public prejudice also played a part in siting—townspeople often objected to the thought of having the mentally ill in their midst, and so built their mental hospitals in completely isolated areas, or near villages which were too small to raise a loud objection.

The normal process of hospitalization is reversed where mental hospitals are concerned; instead of the rural area going to the town for hospitalization, the urban population goes out into the country. Most mental hospitals are situated in areas for which the County Council is the responsible local authority, away from the denser centres of population covered by the county boroughs.

The problem of collaboration is acute in county areas, because of their size, and the scattered nature of population.[1] There may be several mental hospitals within the county boundaries; but many of their patients will come from the county boroughs, which operate separate mental health services. It is often equally acute in large towns for the reverse reason. The hospitals which serve the town may be some miles outside its boundaries. The most satisfactory situation exists in medium-sized county boroughs of comparatively recent growth. A mental hospital may exist within the present boundaries, and have a catchment area which roughly coincides with them. Probably when the hospital was built, it was in a country district, and the town has spread within the last fifty years to surround it. It is no accident that the local authority mental health services which have become well-known since 1948 for efficiency of administration and co-operation with the other branches of the Health Service are in centres of this kind—Nottingham, Oldham,[2] Portsmouth and York spring to mind. Here personal contacts and case conferences have made it possible to obtain a high degree of continuity of care.

The powers and duties of local authorities were set out in the previous chapter. Development has been distinctly uneven, partly because of the difficulties outlined above; partly because of the unequal distribution of social workers, who tend, like most professional people, to prefer to work in large towns, where opportunities for promotion and the development of professional skills are greater; and partly because some Medical Officers of Health do not regard mental health work as a priority.

In a few areas, the initiative in development of after-care services has come from the hospitals, the local authorities continuing to carry out only the statutory duties under the Lunacy and Mental Deficiency Acts. Graylingwell Hospital, near Chichester, has carried out with the consent of the South-west Metropolitan Regional Hospital Board a pilot scheme for psychiatric community service in Worthing and the surrounding area. This involves domiciliary visiting by psychiatrists, out-patient clinics, and a day hospital, all designed as part of an integrated scheme with the aim of keeping patients out of hospital and in the community wherever possible. The Worthing experiment was initiated in 1957, and in 1958, a similar service was developed by the same hos-

[1] A further complication is the practice in County areas of appointing officers who are responsible for a variety of health and welfare services. Mental health work is only a part of their responsibilities.

[2] At Oldham, co-operation is with a psychiatric wing of the General Hospital.

pital in the Chichester area. The Medical Director's report on these two schemes states:

'In this way, the work of the out-patient treatment services and the work of the hospital will dovetail harmoniously, and be providing a psychiatric service meeting the needs of all types of patients . . . as this set-up is essentially a psychiatric service, it would be best for it to be administered and staffed by the parent hospital.'[1]

The North Wales Hospital at Denbigh, which has a well-staffed psychiatric social work department, undertakes after-care in the surrounding area in lieu of the local authorities; and other mental hospitals have assumed varying degrees of responsibility for work of this kind though the intention of section 28 of the National Health Service Act is interpreted elsewhere as placing a clear responsibility on the local authority. The vagueness of section 28 has been in one sense an advantage, since it has enabled local developments to take place with the maximum flexibility in administrative arrangements, as local conditions allow. The fact that patients are adequately cared for is more important than the question of whose responsibility they are.

The Mackintosh Report

The development of local authority work depends largely on the numbers and quality of mental health workers recruited. Dr. Blacker drew attention in 1946 to the fact that the development of community care was likely to be hampered by the shortage of trained social workers in this field.

Within a few days of the appointed day, the Minister of Health set up a committee 'to consider and make recommendations upon questions arising in regard to the supply and demand, training and qualifications of social workers in the Mental Health Service' under the chairmanship of Professor J. M. Mackintosh, Professor of Public Health in the University of London. A report, published in June, 1951, related purely to fully-qualified psychiatric social workers.

By January, 1951, 523 students in all had qualified by means of attendance at a university mental health course. Of these, 331 were then working in the United Kingdom; but only 65 of these were working in mental hospitals, and eight in local authority mental health departments.

---

[1] J. Carse, *The Worthing Experiment*, p. 32.

The rest were divided between out-patient clinics and child guidance work.

The wastage rate was very high. At the London School of Economics in 1949–50, there were 135 applicants, of whom 40 were accepted and only 26 ultimately qualified. The wastage was largely attributable to the fact that the majority of the students were women, many of whom gave up the course, or subsequent employment, on marriage. The Mackintosh Committee estimated that, on a basis of existing training facilities, 65–70 psychiatric social workers could be trained annually. Blacker had said that at least a thousand were needed at once.

Mental Welfare Officers

By 1956, the number of psychiatric social workers in local authority mental health departments had risen from eight to thirty-two; but many local authorities had, for all practical purposes, abandoned the attempt to attract these qualified workers into their employment. The university training departments have, quite rightly, refused to substitute quantity for quality, continuing to select entrants with care and to train them individually. Consequently, the local authorities have had to look elsewhere for their social workers, and other methods of training have had to be considered.

When the new mental health departments of local authorities were set up in 1948, they recruited two very different kinds of workers: Relieving Officers of the Public Assistance Service which had now been superseded by the National Assistance Act 1948, and mental welfare workers from the voluntary associations which had previously been responsible by delegation for the bulk of mental deficiency work in the community.

Until 1948, the Relieving Officer was the person 'duly authorized' under the 1890 Lunacy Act to take proceedings in the case of certification. When the National Assistance Act and the National Health Service Act came into force, some of these men transferred to the employment of the National Assistance Board, whilst others retained their status as 'Duly Authorized Officers' and entered the mental health departments. In most county areas, a form of joint appointment was used, the duly authorized officer also being responsible for welfare services under Part III of the National Assistance Act. Most of the duly authorized officers had an excellent background of work in an administrative setting, but little social work experience, since the previous context of their work had been one in which principles and practice were somewhat rigidly laid down by higher authority.

Under the Mental Deficiency Acts 1913-27, many mental deficiency authorities had delegated their duties to voluntary mental welfare associations, paying the salaries of the associations' workers. Most of these workers were women, many of whom had twenty or thiry years' experience. Their position in 1948 was the reverse of that of the duly authorized officers—they had considerable social work experience—the phrase 'qualified by experience' has a real meaning in social work, where there is much that cannot be learned theoretically, but only by person-to-person contact—but generally little knowledge of the administrative complexities of local authority work.

Both groups have been able, in favourable circumstances, to learn much from each other. In May 1954, the professional associations concerned—the Community Care Section of the Mental Health Worker's Association and the National Association of Duly Authorized Officers —amalgamated, forming the Society of Mental Welfare Officers.

To the older workers transferred in 1948, and to the few psychiatric social workers in the field, younger entrants have been added. Some are graduates in Social Science, who have a wide basic knowledge of the social services in general, though they have little case-work experience, or specialized knowledge of mental health work. Some are qualified mental nurses who have transferred from mental hospitals, preferring the more varied setting offered by community care. Some are local authority clerical workers who have discovered a personal bent for this kind of work, and have transferred from office duties.

A survey undertaken in Lancashire in 1953-4[1] showed that mental health workers in the county area and the seventeen county boroughs came from diverse backgrounds. The total number was 109; of these 36 were previously Relieving Officers, 4 were previously employed by a mental welfare association, 12 (excluding psychiatric social workers) had a degree or a diploma from a university, 14 were trained nurses, and 22 were ex-clerical staff. Only three—employed in Manchester, Liverpool and Oldham—were psychiatric social workers; and 18 had other types of background which were not classifiable.

Outside Liverpool, Manchester, Salford and Oldham, which had highly-organized services, most county boroughs had only two or three mental health workers. The county had 39 for 17 health divisions—an

[1] K. Jones, 'Problems of Mental After-Care in Lancashire'. *Sociological Review*, July, 1954.

average of just over two to each. Few of these workers had clerical assistance, and much time was taken up in typing reports, filing and correspondence. Only one authority regularly provided transport for its workers, and a great deal of time was spent in travelling, particularly in the county divisions, where the workers often had to cover a large rural area with a scattered population by means of very inadequate local 'bus services. Under these conditions, some workers felt that they were only skimming the surface of the work. It was difficult to undertake real case-work, which involves close contact with the patient and his family, or to do preventive work, since so much time was taken up in stemming the flood-tide of urgent, immediate problems. Some workers had gained much from personal contact with psychiatrists who were willing to discuss their problems and give advice. Others felt very isolated—intensely aware of the limitations of their own training, yet unable to find anyone who would give them the help and support they needed.

The Younghusband Report

The Report of the working party on Social Workers in the Local Authority Health and Welfare Services (Younghusband Report)[1] made a number of recommendations which may be expected to affect the staffing position in local authority mental health departments. It is recommended that three types of social workers should be trained and employed:

1. 'Professionally trained and experienced case-workers to undertake case-work in problems of special difficulty.' In the mental health department, this grade would be confined to psychiatric social workers, who would 'have psychiatric consultation, and themselves provide case-work consultation for mental welfare officers'.

2. Officers with a general training in social work, to be provided by the new National Certificate in Social Work. Training for this Certificate would be equivalent to two years' full-time study, and take place outside the universities, mainly in colleges of further education. A bias could be provided in this course for special branches of social work, such as mental health work.

3. Welfare assistants, who would receive planned in-service training, and be able to deal with 'straightforward or obvious needs'.

Salaries should be reviewed, and more senior posts should be made

[1] H.M.S.O., May, 1959.

available. Clerical help and transport should be provided on a much wider scale than is the case. A national council for social work training should be appointed, and a national staff college should be established to give impetus to training and to discussion of social policy in the initial stages.

An outstanding feature of the Younghusband Report is the recognition that workers in many branches of local authority health and welfare work are in fact social workers, and that a common training and a common outlook would greatly ease communication and co-operation between them. As far as the mental health services are concerned, the recommendations of the Report raise several problems which will need further consideration. Mental health work in a local authority is certainly social work; but because of the administrative issues involved, it has other components also. University Departments of Psychiatric Social Work have orientated their courses towards case-work in a psychiatric setting, and have not generally attempted to include training of a kind specifically suitable for local authority work in an already intensive course. The proposal that psychiatric social workers should undertake local authority work in a consultative and supervisory capacity was made in the Mackintosh Report, and is echoed by the Younghusband Committee; but as the Younghusband Report is careful to point out, the ability to act as a consultant and to supervise the work of less highly trained officers is not automatically conferred by a training-course in case-work. Some psychiatric social workers may have this inherent ability, and be able to develop it; others may not. Miss Ashdown and Miss Clement Brown, in their survey of the origin and development of training for psychiatric social work[1] stress the fact that the training is a specialized case-work training, and that the ability to work in an individual and consultative capacity is not an integral part of a psychiatric social worker's professional equipment. Their employment in the kind of capacity envisaged by the Younghusband Report will therefore depend, not only on their professional qualification, but upon personal qualities, and a wide experience of the administrative and legal issues involved in this special form of work. There is at present a great demand for psychiatric social workers who possess these special qualifications, and who are capable of filling senior consultative posts.

The second grade of social workers envisaged is that of workers who have taken the new two-year Certificate in Social Work. Such a course would be of maximum value in providing case-work experience for

[1] Ashdown and Brown, *Social Service and Mental Health*, p. 184.

people with some previous training and experience in mental health work; and it is hoped that local authorities will be able to second existing workers to this course. It seems doubtful whether a two-year course could provide adequate training in social case-work and the special body of knowledge required for mental health departments for new entrants with no previous training or experience.

Welfare assistants are to deal with 'straightforward or obvious needs'; but the Younghusband Committee gives the impression that there will be comparatively little scope for workers of this type in mental health departments, since few of the needs to be met are either straightforward or obvious. It may be possible to use welfare assistants in routine visits to mental defectives of good home background; but even here a sensitive approach is required, and the worker must be able to sense the existence of problems, perhaps unstated and not fully capable of articulate expression, which it is beyond her own capacity to solve.[1] The use of welfare assistants in mental health departments will only be effective under the skilled and sympathetic supervision of more highly qualified workers.

Excluding psychiatric social workers, there were approximately 1,100 social workers in mental health departments. The Younghusband Committee recommended that this number should be doubled, and that these workers should be provided with transport facilities and secretarial help in order to free them from unnecessary delays. These proposals would make it possible to reduce over-heavy case-loads, and would enable workers to concentrate on case-work and prevention more fully.

Financial Problems

The Younghusband Report points the way for future development; but it leaves us, as a report of this nature must, with the practical problems to be solved at local level. Higher salary-scales, improved conditions of work, better prospects for training and promotion, could solve the overall shortage of staff, and attract suitable entrants into a developing profession; but much depends on local initiative and enthusiasm. Some Health Committees, aided and stimulated by their Medical Officers of Health, have regarded the development of a good mental health service as a matter of priority; but in a period when health and welfare services have expanded rapidly, and heavy demands have been made on available resources, other authorities have been

[1] See Mr. Kenneth Robinson's comment on p. 180.

slow to develop their mental health services beyond the minimum statutory requirements.[1] The new system of Treasury grants initiated in 1959,[2] which involves a block grant to local authorities in place of the previous separate grants for each service, gives the local authorities an increased discretion in the allocation of funds. The Mental Health Bill of 1958-9, when first introduced into the House of Commons, provided for a considerable reduction in the statutory requirements to be made on local authorities; and some Members of Parliament feared that, under the block grant system, local authorities might divert money from their mental health service to what they thought were more pressing needs. This fear played a large part in the pressure brought to bear on the Minister of Health to make the provision of preventive and after-care services mandatory.[3] Without regulations from the centre, the service could become more uneven in quality than it is at present.

Like local authorities, mental hospitals have varied considerably in their response to the opportunities of 'the community period'. Some have shown great energy in developing their extramural activities. Some local authorities have appointed a consultant from a near-by hospital as their psychiatric adviser on a sessional basis—a useful link between the two branches of the service. Other consultants are responsible for out-patient clinics, for psychiatric diagnosis and treatment in remand homes, and for work in child guidance clinics. A number of hospitals have made a practice of encouraging members of staff to give talks to outside groups such as Rotary, or Youth Clubs; and of holding 'open days' or arranging conducted tours for interested members of the general public. In these latter activities, there is a double purpose—they increase public understanding on the lines suggested by the Feversham Committee in 1939, and they also help nursing recruitment.

Within the mental hospital itself, the feeling of community has been greatly strengthened. Great advances have been made in clinical, administrative and social psychiatry, of which the full implications are not

---

[1] Lord Feversham stated in the House of Lords (*Hansard*, June 4th, 1959) that 93½ per cent of local authority money spent on the mental health services was spent on the fulfillment of statutory requirements, and only 6½ per cent on prevention and after-care.

[2] Under the Local Government Act, 1958.

[3] The Minister finally agreed to do this under section 28 of the National Health Service Act, 1946. See page. 191.

yet apparent. Techniques of physical treatment—particularly in electro-convulsant therapy and insulin treatment—have been refined. In 1955, the new tranquillizing drugs, of which chlorpromazine and reserpine are perhaps the best known, came into general use. The result has been an astonishing change in the character of mental hospital populations. The duration of stay for acute patients has been appreciably lessened, so that the bulk of new patients now return home within six months of entry into hospital, and many within three months or less.[1] While the total number of admissions has risen from 83,392 in 1955 to 94,020 in 1957, the total number of beds occupied dropped in the same three years by 6,182.[2] There is still a body of long-stay patients—people who have been in mental hospital for years, in whom the hope of recovery and rehabilitation is less; and of psychogeriatric patients, for whom the prognosis is poor; but the introduction of the new drugs has affected these patients too. Increasing numbers are proving capable of a much higher degree of socialization than could previously be expected, and many may be discharged in the future if the community services are able to provide an adequate degree of care for them.

Tranquillizers often make it possible for an agitated patient to be brought under control without being deprived of his liberty or kept under constant surveillance. The repressive features of mental hospital life—locked doors, limitations on parole and patient activities, the custodial role of the mental nurse—have thus lost any sanction they possessed. Hospitals have opened many wards which were previously kept closed. Patient activities have increased, and there is a tendency for the mental hospital to become a busy community rather than a series of locked and largely static segments. Much of the tension which inevitably arose from the fear of violence or the risk of suicide has disappeared.

Work and the Mental Patient

A new interest has been taken in the value of work for the mental patient. In the past, much criticism has been levelled at mental hospitals on the grounds that patients were expected to work at cleaning or in the kitchens or on the farm for the maintenance of the hospital; and that this was a useful means of reducing running costs rather than a means of therapy. One challenge to the old concept of patient-labour came from occupational therapy, which involves the teaching of crafts

---

[1] There is as yet no reliable evidence on the relapse rate.
[2] Annual Reports of Ministry of Health, 1955–7.

and skills in order to arouse interest and activity in the patient, the end-product being comparatively unimportant. A new development is that of the sheltered workshop, where work of commercial value is under-taken—though at a slower pace, and broken down into simpler pro-cesses than in outside industry—and where the patient is paid for his employment. The end-product is important here; but the main aim is to give suitable patients the satisfaction and the experience of something approaching normal working conditions. It may be that occupational therapy is more suited to the acute, short-stay patient, and the sheltered workshop to the stabilized long-stay patient; while there is a case for providing utility work for patients who can be expected to take up domestic or agricultural employment on discharge. Probably all three methods have their value for patients fo differing needs. The important factor is that the work must be suited to the needs of the patient, and undertaken for his benefit.[1]

The 'Therapeutic Community'

The idea of the sheltered workshop is closely linked with new ideas on the social organization of the mental hospital, and the role of the patient within it. The term 'therapeutic community', when applied to mental hospitals, implies a basic orientation in which the community itself becomes the instrument of therapy. A mental patient is an indi-vidual whose social relationships—at home, in employment, in leisure—have been shattered. Part of the process of recovery is learning to live in a small sheltered community which is as far as possible a microcosm of the world outside.

There are two main currents of thought in present-day psychiatry—the 'organic school', which relies for treatment mainly on the tested physical methods, including the new tranquillizing drugs: and the 'psychodynamic school'. Here there is a division between individual psychotherapy, which applies the methods of deep analysis in an exclusive relationship of patient and psychiatrist, and group psycho-therapy, which uses a group situation—possibly a psychiatrist and half a dozen patients—laying stress on the idea of social interaction.[2] The exponents of the ideal of the therapeutic community have drawn heavily on the methods of group psychotherapy, regarding the whole

[1] For a full discussion of this problem, see *The Place of Work in the Treatment of Mental Disorder*, Report of N.A.M.H. Conference, 1959.

[2] See, *inter al.*, S. H. Foulkes and E. S. Anthony, *Group Psychotherapy*, *passim*. Foulkes, 'Group Analysis', *Lancet*, March 2nd, 1946.

mental hospital community as the group, but their methods are generally less intensive than those of the psychoanalytic school.

'Briefly,' writes Dr. Maxwell Jones of the Industrial Neurosis Unit at Belmont Hospital,

'we attempt to absorb the patient into the Unit community, which has developed a definite culture of its own. This culture . . . is maintained and perpetuated through the staff rather than through the patients, though in practice it is difficult to separate these two groups in the community. Educational techniques, mainly in the form of discussion groups, seem to aid any change in social attitudes in the desocialized patient. As far as possible, social and vocational roles are provided for him while still in hospital. . . . These roles approximate as far as possible to what is found in the relatively healthy outside community.'[1]

To some extent, this is the re-discovery of an old idea; for community life has always been a feature of mental hospital organizations, and the early, small asylums were often therapeutic communities in a generalized sense; but the sheer pressure of numbers in the late nineteenth century meant the loss of human values and personal relationships. The methods of social psychiatry have led to a renewed emphasis on the personal and social aspects of administration and therapy.

'The time has come,' states a medical officer from Cheadle Royal Hospital,

'. . . when we have to recognize that the patients' individuality must be preserved even while in hospital. Patients should be trusted. They should have as much responsibility for running their life as they can, participating in ward committees, organizing self-government, and having no mean say in the working of any organization of the hospital in which they reside. . . . Since the patient is being trained to return to the outside community, the hospital should resemble this outside community as nearly as it can. Every way in which the hospital diverges from that outside must be scrutinized: and under this scrutiny, many of the old restrictive asylum practices—locked doors, sharp tools forbidden, no matches, no razors, no mixing of the sexes—are seen to be unnecessary . . . hostility should be met with patience; violence with restraint, but not with anger; childishness with understanding; and feeble attempts at independence with encouragement.'[2]

[1] M. Jones, *Social Psychiatry*, p. xv.
[2] The Therapeutic Community—Mental Patients and Staffs, *Manchester Guardian*, January 29th, 1959.

Three factors—the use of new tranquillizing drugs, the new freedom of movement and activity implied by the open door and the increased use of parole, the concept of the therapeutic community—have revolutionized mental hospital life in the past few years. To some extent they are interdependent, though the emphasis varies from hospital to hospital. They imply a new status for the mental patient, in which his individuality is preserved, and he is treated as retaining the capacity for initiative and for some degree of responsibility. They require a high level of adaptability and psychiatric skill in mental hospital staff. Particularly important in this respect are the role of the medical superintendent and the role of the mental nurse, both of which involve controversial and difficult issues.

The Medical Superintendent

Mental hospitals and mental deficiency hospitals, like tuberculosis and fever hospitals, have retained medical superintendents since 1948. Other hospitals have not. The National Health Service Act emphasized by implication the lay administration of general hospitals, since the hospital secretary became secretary to the Management Committee,[1] and the Committee's chief officer. The position of the medical superintendent in mental hospitals was specifically safeguarded by the National Health Service (Superintendents of Mental Hospitals) Regulations, 1948.[2] Hospital secretaries in mental hospitals have been loth to accept second place, and, in a unified Health Service, have tended to claim the position of authority which would be theirs in other hospitals. Medical superintendents have tended to defend what they regard as a primarily psychiatric sphere against the incursion of lay administrators. The result has sometimes been a conflict in role-playing played out in terms of personalities, in which professional pride has been roused on both sides.

The case for lay administration of mental hospitals was put by Mr. J. Crawford Field at the Institute of Public Administration's Conference on the Health Service in 1951 in the following terms:

'A hospital is a multi-craft organization. . . . There is a feeling in some people's minds that because in a hospital so many of the important people are doctors, a doctor should be 'at the head' . . . the office of

---

[1] In teaching hospitals, the officer of comparable status is usually the House Governor, who is secretary to the Board of Governors.

[2] A few general hospitals, and all isolation and tuberculosis hospitals, have also retained the post of Medical Superintendent.

medical superintendent as hospital administrator represents a mistaken policy, because it breaks the rule of giving each craft equal consideration. . . .'[1]

In 1951, the Institute of Hospital Administrators produced a report in which a claim was made for the introduction of lay administration in mental hospitals. In a section headed 'Potential Interference', this report stated, 'There are no arguments to justify the continued existence of a separate system, built upon principles of medical administration, for the mental hospital services.' The main arguments against medical administration developed here were that it made for considerable difficulties in administration in mixed groups of hospitals, where the group secretary's role demanded that he should have equal control over all the hospitals in the group; that medical superintendents tended to have excessive influence with Hospital Management Committees.

Against these arguments, it has been contended that mental hospitals, because of their community organization, represent a special case. If the community is the instrument of therapy, then the therapist must be in charge. The Third Report of the World Health Organization's Expert Committee states:

'The creation of the milieu of the therapeutic community, and the fostering of the relationships and activities which compose it, are the therapeutic task of the medical director. It is for this reason that the therapeutic community can never be created under the direction of a lay administrator. It is in essence a technical psychiatric task.'[2]

If the methods of social psychiatry have a future, the position of the medical superintendent is clearly of crucial importance. If, on the other hand, the bulk of present mental health work moves out into the community services, and the mental hospital becomes an institution used only for deteriorated long-stay patients to be treated by organic methods, the need for psychiatric supervision of the hospital community may disappear, and the medical superintendent's place be taken by a lay administrator without loss of clinical efficiency. The future depends largely on research and experimentation within psychiatry itself.[3]

[1] *The Health Services: Some of their Practical Problems*, Institute of Public Administration, 1951.
[2] W.H.O. Technical Report Series No.73, 1953, p. 19.
[3] The National Health Service (Superintendents of Mental Hospitals) Regulations, 1948, will be revoked when the main provisions of the Mental Health Act 1959 come into force. Contractual rights of existing superintendents will be safeguarded. (*Lancet* May 14th 1960.)

Whatever view one takes of the professional claims made on both sides in this controversy, it is clear that continuation of the controversy is not in the best interests of the mental hospital service. Perhaps the test of administrative talent in both lay and medical administrators is their ability to work with each other.

The position of the medical superintendent has also been affected in relation to his medical colleagues. Traditionally in psychiatry, medical administration as distinct from clinical practice has carried a special status and high financial rewards. Dr. Blacker pointed out in *Neurosis and the Mental Health Services* that the assumption that an administrative post was the crown of a psychiatrist's career often entailed a waste of clinical skill, since prospects for clinicians were poor, and a good clinician did not necessarily make a first-class administrator. The National Health Service improved the position of the clinical psychiatrist by introducing a system of grading in which the senior rank was that of consultant. The medical superintendent, though carrying out duties which are different in function from those of other psychiatrists in his hospital, and which involve some degree of non-clinical supervision over them, has the same status and salary as those of his staff who have reached consultant status. The post of medical superintendent is thus no longer the crown of a career, since a psychiatrist can reach a position of the same eminence without forfeiting his clinical work, and without assuming heavy administrative responsibilities. As Blacker hoped, men of high ability have been preserved in this way for clinical psychiatry; but the position of the medical superintendent has been complicated with respect to his senior colleagues; and fewer men of high calibre have been willing to take on the burdens of administration.

The Mental Nurse

The role of the mental nurse is also much under discussion at present. In the past, the main work of the nursing staff in a mental hospital has been custodial in character. It involved keeping patients clean and fed, making sure that they did not escape, or do harm to themselves or to other people. Today, a much higher degree of skill and personal adaptability is required of the good psychiatric nurse, who must learn to know the patient as a human being undergoing a process of development rather than as a 'case' to be guarded and cared for. Yet, while the demands on the mental nurse are such that they can only be satisfied by people of intelligence and a high degree of personal integration, there is an acute shortage of trained and qualified staff.[1] Many hospitals are so short of nursing staff, trained or untrained, that they are in no position to lay down qualifications of any kind for employment. Recruitment campaigns have been initiated, and some hospitals have appointed nurses from abroad, bringing over applicants from Ireland, France, Italy, Spain and the West Indies. This is a temporary solution only in the majority of cases, since few of these nurses wish to spend their whole working lives in England, and many return to their own countries after qualifying.

Mental nursing still does not carry the same prestige as general nursing, and has never been a popular profession. The number of people with a real vocation to the work is not enough to fill the many vacancies; and in a period of full employment, there are more attractive kinds of employment available, many of which offer higher wages, shorter hours, and less responsibility. There was a high level of recruitment, particularly among male nurses, during the economic depression of the nineteen-thirties, and many who came to the mental hospitals in search of a steady and pensionable job remained, and made excellent nurses, when there were other forms of work to be had. These nurses are now in the last ten years of their working life, and when they retire, a serious situation will become acute.

The *Lancet* has commented, 'Standards in our mental hospitals are now very low, and unless the nursing crisis is handled successfully, they are in danger of falling to the level from which such men as Tuke reclaimed them.'[2]

The Manchester Mental Nursing Survey, published in 1955, suggested that a solution to the shortage of trained staff might be found by a redistribution of work among the available grades of staff, greater use being made of less highly skilled workers than the Registered Mental Nurse for routine work. As far as the overall shortage of all workers was concerned, the report of the Survey suggested the discontinuation of the 'long day' system (that is, one day shift and one night shift to cover twenty-four hours) in favour of the three-shift system, which involves a shorter day but less complete free days. It also recommended an increase in the employment of part-time nurses, of whom married female nurses are the most readily available. Since the publication of this report,

[1] The Royal-Medico-Psychological Association agreed to cease separate examining in 1946, and the last R.M.P.A. examination was held in 1951. A new and experimental G.N.C. syllabus for mental nurses, drafted largely by the R.M.P.A. and approved by both bodies, was introduced in 1958.

[2] *Lancet*, December 13th, 1947.

most mental hospitals have transferred to the three-shift system. Employment of part-time nurses varies according to local needs and availability. It is most used in hospitals in rural areas, where there are few other forms of work for married women, and least where there is an industrial centre within easy daily reach.

. . . . .

Mental hospitals have many problems, but the general picture today is one of activity and development, with varied possibilities. This is in itself an achievement in a sphere where, for nearly a hundred years, there was little progress and much apathy.

OUT-PATIENT CLINICS

Dr. Blacker's survey in 1946 showed that there was a marked disparity in the provision of psychiatric out-patient facilities. Doctor-sessions per week per million population amounted to 26·7 in London, and to only 4·9 in Wales. There were 3·74 clinics per million population in the north of England, but more than twice as many in the south. A questionnaire was sent to 216 clinics, and an 86 per cent response was obtained. This showed that for every ten clinics in voluntary hospitals, there were two in municipal hospitals and only one in a mental hospital. Some of the clinics had elaborate records, but others were unable to answer the questionnaire because they had no permanent records at all. In several, the practice was for the doctor to make brief notes while talking to the patient, to telephone the report to the patient's family doctor, and then to tear up his notes. Here was a poor basis for continuity of care.

Clinics in voluntary hospitals usually dealt only with neurotic patients. They had more frequent sessions than the others, and better-qualified staff. Clinics in mental hospitals, or attached to mental hospitals, dealt largely with psychotic patients, had less frequent sessions, but were generally better equipped with psychiatric social workers.

The atmosphere and procedure in clinics varied enormously. Some were cheerful places where the patient was seen by appointment, made to feel at home, interviewed and examined in pleasant surroundings, and treated with courtesy. Others were 'draughty, ill-lit and forbidding'. A patient might be kept waiting for one or two hours and be seen by a hurried and preoccupied doctor. In these circumstances, it was doubtful whether the visit could achieve much, or whether the patient would return.

The directory of adult psychiatric out-patient facilities in England and Wales published by the National Association for Mental Health in 1957 lists over eight hundred out-patient clinics. Many have psychiatric social workers attached, and secretarial help. No information is available concerning the total number of cases dealt with by these clinics, nor the facilities offered by them, but it can be said in general that the standard of provision has risen considerably under the Health Service, and that the volume of work covered—pre-care, after-care and care as an alternative to hospitalization—is still expanding rapidly. Some clinics now offer a wide range of facilities, including physical treatments and occupational therapy. It is not possible to draw more than an artificial distinction between clinics of this type and day hospitals. Most psychiatric consultants now spend two or three sessions a week on out-patient work.

DAY HOSPITALS AND NIGHT HOSPITALS

As the mental hospital approaches more closely in its organization to the life of the community outside, and the community assumes, through the local authority services, a new responsibility for the care of the mentally ill and mental defectives, there have been several experiments which seek to bridge the gap between the two. In the mental deficiency field, hostels have for many years enabled stabilized defectives who lack a suitable home to live with some care and supervision, going out each day to a simple form of employment, such as unskilled agricultural labour; since the introduction of the National Health Service, local authorities and mental deficiency hospitals have both been able to develop such hostels, either separately or by joint action. Some mental hospitals have a few patients who go out to work during the day, using the hospital as a 'night hospital' only; but there are many more stabilized patients who do not need the full resources of the hospital, though they are not able to return home because of domestic or personal difficulties. The development of 'half-way houses' or 'night hospitals' for such patients, who are capable of making a limited contribution to the community if provided with minimal nursing and medical care, is widely recognized as necessary and desirable. To date, it has been hampered by the administrative divisions of the Health Service—since this is a field of development which does not clearly belong either to the hospital or the local authority—and by restrictions on capital expenditure.

A different problem is that of the patient who needs treatment or nursing care during the day, but who can return to his own home at night. Given a good home background, the patient's needs may be better served by day treatment than by total hospitalization. At present, more than forty day hospitals are in operation, dealing in all with some 1,500 patients. Some cater for psychogeriatric patients, and provide only nursing care and occupational therapy. Others cater for acute short-stay patients who are able to live at home, and offer a wide range of treatment including physical treatments and group and individual psychotherapy. Most of the centres opened so far are small, taking from eight to thirty patients. Some are only able to take patients once or twice a week. With a few exceptions, day hospitals have been initiated by the hospital branch of the Health Service, though not always by mental hospitals—general hospitals and university departments of psychiatry have played a part in this development.

Whether day hospitals are less expensive than the normal psychiatric hospital, and whether they in fact require less staff, is still debatable. It is possible that transport costs will prove so high that they offset the saving in the provision of night accommodation; and that an effective day hospital requires a team of social workers whose recruitment is more difficult and more expensive than that of night staff; but whatever the financial issues involved, there is clearly a place for the day hospital on purely social grounds, since this form of organization provides the means whereby some patients can retain a link with their own homes while receiving mental treatment. From the clinical point of view, this may be a distinct advantage, since the patient does not have to adapt to mental hospital conditions and then re-adapt to home conditions again at a later date.

THE NATIONAL ASSOCIATION FOR MENTAL HEALTH

The assumption of responsibility for community care by the statutory authorities has not led to the end of voluntary activity, but rather to an increase in the influence of the National Association. Since its formation in November, 1946, it has worked in partnership with the Ministry of Health and the Board of Control, organizing training courses, sponsoring public enlightenment campaigns, and organizing professional conferences. At a local level, its local associations continue to find ways and means of supplementing the statutory services. The distinctive contribution of a voluntary agency in the field of social service is its ability to adapt continually to meet new needs, to fill gaps in the existing service, and to rally public opinion. The National Association for Mental Health has shown its capacity for fulfilling these functions, and has justified the Feversham Committee's recommendation for the unification of voluntary effort.

The *Lancet* commented in 1948 that there was an unevenness about the growth of N.A.M.H. There was a great increase in the demand for talks about mental health, but comparatively little money was forthcoming to support its work. The general public had accepted the idea of mental health work intellectually, but was resisting it emotionally:

'It is easy enough to say "poor feller" when the amnesic hero of a film reveals his mental anguish in appropriately moving gestures: much harder to bear at close quarters the difficult old aunt who hides rubbish in drawers and looks so odd to the people next door. . . .'

Helping the public to an emotional acceptance of mental health problems is perhaps the special task of the National Association.

. . . .

The general trend since 1948 has been for the development of a community service operating in a number of different ways to meet a variety of social and clinical needs. Domiciliary visits, social after-care, out-patient clinics, day hospitals, night hospitals, half-way houses—all play a part which is complementary to that of the hospital. The World Health Organization's Expert Committee contrasts the 'classical' concept of psychiatric services—in which the hospital is the basic unit, and all other services are seen as extensions of the hospital's function—with the 'modern' concept, in which a medico-social team is responsible 'for all the mental health problems of the community and . . . the psychiatric hospital . . . one of many tools for carrying out its work'.[1] Present administrative difficulties and professional interests may divide the team. It is not easy for local authorities to work together with hospitals, or for workers with different forms of training and different orientation to collaborate; but if the reality is still far off, at least the ideal of the community mental health service has won wide acceptance.

[1] W.H.O. Technical Report Series No. 73, 1953, p. 37.

This chapter has been concerned with main trends of development, and with some of the problems and experiments of the period since the National Health Service came into being. It is now necessary to go back to 1954 in order to trace the immediate growth of the movement which led to the Mental Health Act.

Chapter Twelve

THE MENTAL HEALTH ACT, 1959

AT the beginning of 1954, there had been no major revision and consolidation of the lunacy code for sixty-four years: for the Act of 1890, though to some extent by-passed by the 1930 Mental Treatment Act and the Mental Deficiency Acts 1913–27, was still in force. It was over a quarter of a century since the Macmillan Commission had recommended sweeping changes, and many of the recommendations of that commission had not yet been put into practice. There had not been a full-dress parliamentary debate on mental health since February 17th, 1930, when the Rt. Hon. Arthur Greenwood, as Minister of Health, spoke on the Mental Treatment Bill.

On October 22nd 1953, the appointment was announced of a Royal Commission 'On the Law Relating to Mental Illness and Mental Deficiency'. From this time dates a tremendous increase in public interest in mental health problems which coincided with the clinical and social progress outlined in the previous chapter. In February of the following year, the membership of the Royal Commission was announced; and a parliamentary debate lasting five hours opened the subject to public discussion.

The Parliamentary Debate of February 19th, 1954

The debate was initiated by Mr. Kenneth Robinson, Labour Member of Parliament for St. Pancras North, who had a personal interest in mental health for some years, and had become chairman of the north-west Metropolitan Regional Hospital's Board's Mental Health Committee in 1952. The terms of the motion set the tone for the debate which followed:

'That this House, whilst recognizing the advances made in recent years in the treatment and care of mental patients, expresses its concern at the serious overcrowding of mental hospitals and mental deficiency hospitals, and at the acute shortage of nursing and junior medical staff in the Mental Health Service; and calls upon H.M. Government and the hospital authorities to make adequate provision for the modernization and development of this essential service.'

He stressed that this was not a party matter. He had no wish to make political capital out of the deficiencies which he was about to outline.

'There are shortcomings, many shortcomings, but they are not the responsibility of any particular Government; they are the responsibility of numerous successive Governments, and of the local authorities as well, and are perhaps due even more to public apathy and ignorance.'

After paying tribute to the advances which had taken place in the medical and social fields, and mentioning the impending appointment of a Royal Commission which would consider 'the out of date and unsatisfactory state of the law', Mr. Robinson went on to direct attention to four main shortages: shortage of beds,[1] shortage of suitable buildings, shortage of staff, and shortage of money.

There was serious overcrowding in many mental hospitals. Sometimes the patients were crowded together, their beds no more than nine inches apart. Sometimes beds were placed in the corridors; and still there were not enough beds. This meant that patients were often kept on a waiting list for long periods, and their condition deteriorated till they were sometimes beyond treatment when they were finally admitted.

The figures for discharges from mental hospital were largely illusory. A hospital of 2,000 beds might show a discharge rate of 1,000 per annum. This did not mean that the average length of stay could be reasonably estimated at two years. It meant that a small number of short-stay beds had a rapid turnover—patients changing every few weeks. The rest of the beds were filled by chronic patients who stayed many years. There was no evidence that, with all the advances in treatment, the rate of chronicity was dropping. In fact, we had an ageing population, and it might well be increasing.

In mental deficiency, the position was even worse. The ascertained

---

[1] This debate took place before the developments referred to in the previous chapter which have begun to reduce the overall demand on beds since 1955.

waiting list for mental deficiency beds in the country as a whole was 9,000, of whom nearly half were children, many low-grade defectives.

'I want the House to reflect on what the existence of one of these low-grade defectives means in a family ... somebody in the family, usually the mother who is perhaps harassed with several other young children, has got to be constantly cleaning up after this child, keeping a constant eye on it to see that it does not injure itself or set fire to the house or do some damage ... this means an intolerable strain.... This situation causes untold misery, and every one of these defectives in a family means that the lives of two, three or half a dozen other people must be affected adversely.'

Not only was there an overall shortage of accommodation, but most of the accommodation which existed was unsuitable, since the hospitals had been built to fit an outmoded concept of what mental illness and mental deficiency were:

'The Victorians could not build other than solidly, and there the buildings stand, grim, almost indestructible, and they constitute the majority of our mental hospital accommodation.'

Regional Hospital Boards faced a dilemma of considerable dimensions: should they spend their limited resources on trying to patch up these 'really hopeless buildings'? What most of them had done was to develop small modern units for short-stay patients; but the chronic long-stay patients remained in the 'institutional atmosphere of these Victorian barracks'.

Mr. Robinson went on to discuss the serious repercussions of the nursing shortage. In his own region alone, there were 58 vacancies for trained mental nurses, and 508 vacancies for other nurses. Between 200 and 250 beds were closed for lack of staff. He pressed for a new recognition of the professional role of the mental nurse, a new grade of mental nurses with a simpler and less theoretical training than that needed for the qualification of Registered Mental Nurse, the extension of the cadet schemes for young people between school-leaving age and eighteen, and for a national Press and poster campaign which would put the issues squarely before the public.

Shortage of money was at the root of many troubles. The Medical Research Council had spent nearly eight million pounds on research in eight years, but of this sum only a little over one per cent had been spent on research into mental health—despite the fact that mental patients occupied 42 per cent of all hospital beds.[1] Out of the total of forty million pounds' capital expenditure in the first five years of the Health Service, only 16 per cent had been spent on mental hospitals. The Minister had set aside a million pounds for the coming year specially for capital development in mental hospitals and mental deficiency institutions,

'. . . but he knows, and we all know, that this is a drop in the ocean. We want many, many millions, and we want them urgently.'

Mr. Robinson's last words were an echo of Ashley's words in the parliamentary debate which preceded the passing of the 1845 Lunatics Act:

'These people are a small minority with no voice with which to speak, and most of them without the vote. That is all the more reason why we in this House should see to it that they are getting the best which we can give.'[2]

Subsequent speakers took up the points which had been raised, and contributed many examples from their own experience, or that of their constituents, which illustrated the pressing need for action. Dr. Somerville Hastings (Barking) and Mr. J. K. Vaughan-Morgan (Reigate) challenged the statement concerning the need for more hospital beds, pointing out that modern trends were towards increasing community care, and thereby relieving the pressure on existing beds. Mr. R. J. Mellish (Bermondsey) stated that the average cost per patient per week in a general hospital, according to the Ministry of Health's costing returns for 1953, was £13 3s. 6d. The comparable figure for mental hospitals was £4 6s. 7d. and for mental deficiency hospitals £4 1s. 7d. Although mental institutions had some means of cutting down maintenance costs—the patients produced some of their own food, and provided labour for unskilled tasks—he felt that this great disparity was unjustified.

Miss Hornsby-Smith, Parliamentary Secretary to the Ministry of Health, replied for the Government. She expressed thanks to Mr. Robinson for 'taking the opportunity to initiate an outstanding and

---

[1] Since the duration of stay in hospital is longer in mental hospitals, they represented only 3 per cent of all admissions; but even so, the figure for expenditure on research was disproportionately low.

[2] Ashley's speech ended, 'These unhappy persons are outcasts from all the social and domestic affections of private life, and have no refuge but in the laws . . . the motion is made on behalf of the most helpless, if not the most afflicted, portion of the human race.'

valuable debate . . . and for refusing to be persuaded by his hon. Friends to talk about gambling instead'. She did not think that the volume of mental illness or mental deficiency as such were increasing; but people were living longer—which increased the number of psychogeriatric patients—and the new outlook on mental illness meant that people were willing to come forward more readily for treatment on a voluntary basis. She agreed that existing buildings were 'an appalling legacy'; but pointed out that replacing them was 'not a question of a few million pounds . . . (but) a question of thousands of millions over many years'.

The motion was put, and agreed to by the House.

The value of this debate lay less in the facts which emerged—for all these facts were well-known to people working in the mental health field—than in the impetus which it gave to a public movement for reform. It aroused the public conscience (it was well reported by the Press) and put the Government of the day on its mettle. Mental health became a burning public issue. The debate provided an excellent curtain-raiser to the more lengthy and specialized work of the Royal Commission.

THE ROYAL COMMISSION ON MENTAL ILLNESS AND MENTAL DEFICIENCY

The full terms of reference of the Commission were as follows:

'To inquire, as regards England and Wales, into the existing law and administrative machinery governing the certification, detention, care (other than hospital care or treatment under the National Health Service Acts, 1946–52), absence on trial or licence, discharge and supervision of persons who are or are alleged to be suffering from mental illness or mental defect, other than Broadmoor patients; to consider, as regards England and Wales, the extent to which it is now, or should be made, statutorily possible for such persons to be treated as voluntary patients, without certification; and to make recommendations.'

Though the discussions later recorded in the Minutes of Evidence were to range over a wide field, the Commission was thus limited to legal and administrative issues, with a clear directive to the effect that they were to consider ways of reducing the existing formalities of admission and discharge, and ways of extending community care. They were concerned only with what the law could do, not with the wider issues of public attitudes and prejudices, with clinical matters, or with the pressing and immediate problems of shortage.

The members appointed to the Royal Commission included such eminent names as Sir Russell Brain in the neurological field, and Dr. T. P. Rees, then medical superintendent of Warlingham Park Hospital, in psychiatry. The chairman was Lord Percy, who, as Lord Eustace Percy, had served for a short time on the Royal Commission of 1926. Lady Adrian[1] had a distinguished record of voluntary service in the mental health field. Mrs. Braddock had a wide knowledge of both parliamentary and local authority procedure, plus a rare and valuable energy. Other members were Sir Cecil Oakes, a member of the Central Health Services Council; Mr. Claude Bartlett, a male nurse, and President of the Confederation of Health Service Employees; Mr. Hylton-Foster, Q.C., later the Solicitor-General; Mr. R. M. Jackson, an eminent jurist; Dr. Howell Thomas, medical superintendent of Cell Barnes Mental Deficiency Hospital, and Dr. J. G. Wilson, Medical Officer of Health for the Port and City of London.

The Royal Commission, in a period of just over three years, received memoranda of evidence from 68 associations, societies, local authorities, hospital authorities or Government departments; and from 250 individual persons, including people professionally engaged in mental health work, patients, patients' relatives, and former patients. They received oral evidence from 42 associations and 11 individuals, most of this evidence being taken in public. Many professional bodies drew up memoranda, some of them covering the entire range of mental health work, for the Commission's consideration. Out of this mass of evidence, covering all possible shades of opinion, and often expressing contradictory points of view, the Royal Commission drew up a report of a little over three hundred pages which summarized the main problems and the main trends of public opinion, and provided a blue-print for a comprehensive mental health service. The written style is a little laborious, and the Report lacks the clarity, the sudden vivid and memorable phrases, which characterized its predecessor of 1926; but this may be due to a change in the subject-matter. Issues which appeared simple and clear-cut in 1926 were seen to be many-sided in 1957; and mental health is now too complex a subject, with too great a weight of material, for vivid, simple writing.

[1] Wife of the Master of Trinity College, Cambridge, and daughter of Dame Ellen Pinsent (q.v.).

The main recommendations of the Report were as follows:[1]

1. *A New Legal Terminology*

In future, the basic term 'mental disorder' should be used to cover all forms of mental ill-health. Three main categories of persons suffering from 'mental disorder' should be recognized:

      (*a*) 'mentally ill patients';
      (*b*) 'psychopathic patients';
      (*c*) 'severely subnormal patients'.

These changes in terminology implied considerable changes in principle. The use of a single term which covered both mental illness and mental deficiency involved the belief that these two conditions, though medically and socially very different from one another, could be treated as one in law. The legal issues involved were the same, and one Act of Parliament could provide for both. Previously, as we have seen, legislation for mentally ill patients (the Lunacy and Mental Treatment Acts) and that for mental defectives (the Mental Deficiency Acts) have run on separate, though often parallel, lines.

The replacement of the phrase 'patients of unsound mind' by 'mentally ill patients' is largely a matter of euphemism, of finding a phrase more acceptable to present-day thought. The Report made it clear that this category should include old people whose mental disorder was attributable to organic changes, though the Commission had been under some pressure to remove them from the scope of the mental health services altogether.

'Psychopathic patients' were recognized as a separate category for the first time. No attempt was made to frame a legal definition of psychopathy, and the question of defining this group of persons suffering from character disorders was left to the medical profession.[2]

'Severely subnormal patients' involved a new attitude to mental deficiency. This term was to cover idiots and imbeciles as defined in the existing Mental Deficiency Acts, and those feeble-minded patients incapable of leading an independent life. No legal provisions were envisaged for feeble-minded persons able to maintain themselves in the community.

[1] A discussion of the Minutes of Evidence and a fuller outline of recommendations is given in Appendix III.
[2] See p. 214 for a medical definition quoted in the Minutes of Evidence of the Royal Commission.

2. *Administration*

The Board of Control was to be abolished. Its functions as an inspectorate would be taken over by the Ministry of Health, which could consider the total psychiatric resources of an area rather than treating the mental hospitals in isolation. Its functions as a body to which appeals could be made against compulsory detention in individual cases would be taken over by Mental Health Review Tribunals—new bodies constituted on a local basis in each Regional Hospital Board area.

The Royal Commission endorsed the wisdom of the decision to integrate the mental health services with the general health and welfare services, implemented under the National Health Service Act of 1946. They considered that integration should be increased. This was a clear swing away from the earlier policy of creating special organizations to deal with mental health needs. It was recommended that where possible, the education department should deal with severely subnormal children, the welfare services with mentally infirm old people. In each case, the mental health department, or the mental hospital, should only be involved as a last resort.

The special designation of mental hospitals, which prevented them from taking other types of patient, and prevented certified mental patients from entering other hospitals, should cease. Hospitals should be able to specialize, but as in the case of other forms of illness, specialization should be a matter of administrative and medical arrangement, not of legal requirement.

3. *Admission and Discharge*

Patients should be admitted to mental hospitals and mental deficiency hospitals as to other types of hospital—without special formalities of any kind. Certification—now termed 'compulsory detention'—would be used only where treatment was deemed urgently necessary, and where informal treatment was refused. Most patients would be admitted freely—and would be able to discharge themselves at any time. These proposals replaced the much more limited provisions for voluntary and temporary treatment under the Mental Treatment Act 1930, and introduced a new concept in mental deficiency legislation, where all admission had previously been under a compulsory order, and the initiative in securing discharge had to come from the hospital authorities.

The recommended procedures in cases where compulsion is necessary are developed from those in use at the time of the Report under the Lunacy Act, 1890—admission for observation (limit, twenty-eight days), admission for treatment, and emergency admission (limit, seventy-two hours). A striking factor here is the abolition of the magistrate's order, introduced among so much controversy in the eighteen-eighties. Two medical certificates would be required to support a petition from a relative of a mental welfare officer of the local authority. Patients might also be placed under compulsory guardianship.

Special procedures were outlined for use where a psychopathic patient was involved. For an adult psychopath—over twenty-one—compulsory detention could only be secured for the four-week period of an observation order. A psychopath might be compulsorily detained for treatment under the age of twenty-one, and could then be detained until he reached the age of twenty-five.

4. Mental Health Review Tribunals

New bodies, organized on a regional basis, should take over from the Board of Control the duty of investigating cases of alleged wrongful detention, and patients should have access to these tribunals at specified times.

THE MENTAL HEALTH BILL IN THE COMMONS

The Mental Health Bill was published, and had its first reading, in December, 1958. The second reading was introduced in the Commons by the Minister of Health, Mr. Derek Walker-Smith, on January 26th, 1959. He pointed out that the Bill was a long one—it contained 146 clauses and eight separate schedules—but that it replaced in comparatively simple form a mass of legislation, repealing fifteen whole Acts, and thirty-seven Acts in part. He referred to *The Times*, which had called the existing laws on mental health 'a jungle'.

'They are certainly complex, difficult, and in many respects out of date. Consequently, in replacing the mosaic—to use a politer term—of the law and procedure produced by our fathers and forefathers, with a single contemporary design, we are making a clean sweep. But this holocaust of the laws made by our predecessors does not carry any condemnation of their actions. They, particularly in the nineteenth and early twentieth century, laboured for progress in their day as we do in ours. . . .'

The existing laws had been good in their day; but advances in medical and social skills, a new change in public attitudes 'as rapid as it is welcome' had rendered them out of date. In the new Bill, two principles had been followed: the provision of as much treatment as possible on a voluntary and informal basis; and a new system of safeguards where compulsion must continue to be used, which would attempt to draw anew the line between the liberty of the subject and the protection of society.

The Minister outlined the provisions of the Bill, touching particularly on points at which it diverged from the recommendations of the Royal Commission. To the three categories of patients—mentally ill, psychopathic, severely subnormal—a fourth, subnormal, had been added.[1] A definition of psychopathy had been attempted, involving three factors: a persistent disorder of personality, 'abnormally aggressive or seriously irresponsible conduct', and susceptibility to medical treatment. Although the Royal Commission had recommended that the Minister of Health should be given an overriding power of discharge in the case of patients compulsorily detained, the Bill did not give him this power, because it was felt that the exercise of such a power would detract from the standing and authority of the new Mental Health Review Tribunals. The Minister could, however, refer a case to a Tribunal at any time. (The times at which cases could normally be referred to Tribunals were otherwise limited by the Act.)

'One of the main principles we are seeking to pursue,' said the Minister, 'is the re-orientation of the mental health services away from institutional care towards care in the community.' The mental health services of local authorities, judging from expenditure, were expanding rapidly. In 1954-5, their cost was a little over £2¼ million. In 1957-8, it was over £3½ million; and in 1958-9, it was estimated that it would increase again by half a million pounds, to over £4 million.

The Royal Commission had recommended that there should be a specific grant for capital development by local authorities. The Minister admitted that this had not been possible, and also that the grant to the mental health services was now part of the general grant. This was, whether members liked it or not, a *fait accompli*. 'We cannot debate the issue of the general grant all over again in the course of this Bill.'

---

[1] Under the Royal Commission's fairly stringent definition of 'severely subnormal', a large number of feeble-minded persons might have been suddenly released into the community without adequate care.

Although he felt that the principles of the Bill were right, he wished to keep an open mind as to details:

'When we come to Committee, we shall come with no obstinate pride of authorship. We shall listen to suggestions, animated by the desire to make this as good a Bill as our corporate wisdom can achieve. ... On the Statute Book, it will mark a notable chapter in the history of social progress, and reflect credit on the Parliament which enacts it.'

Dr. Summerskill, in a long speech, took up the question of the general grant. She regarded it as 'deplorable' as far as the mental health services were concerned:

'How can the right hon. and learned gentleman on the one hand commend to the House the proposals of the Royal Commission, which we all applaud, and on the other ignore the practical recommendations of the Royal Commission? The Commission was composed of sensible and practical people who knew that it was stupid to expound this great ideal to the people and at the same time refrain from allowing them to have sufficient money to put it into operation.'

Sir Hugh Lucas-Tooth was concerned about the split between hospital care and local authority care. The boundary problem, in its present form, seemed insoluble; but gradually the large old hospitals were to be broken up, and he felt that the most acceptable solution was to site small hospitals, where possible, to fit in with local authority areas.

Several members continued the discussion about local authority services. Mr. Christopher Mayhew sounded a sober note: 'What matters is not passing the Bill, but what comes after it.' The record of the local authorities 'with certain spectacular exceptions' had not been encouraging to date. He endorsed the suggestion of Mr. Kenneth Robinson that local authorities should be required to put forward their plans for development over the next two years. The Bill, though it described the powers of local authorities in more detail, in fact added nothing to the powers they already possessed under section 28 of the National Health Service Act. They could do a great deal; but they were actually required to do very little.

Mr. Mayhew urged the House to think carefully about the matter of community care. A great deal of lip-service was paid to the idea of getting patients out into the community again, but this was not a simple matter. There was a good deal of public prejudice to be overcome; and quite apart from prejudice, there were deeper problems:

'We shall not get anywhere unless we realize frankly that, by the very nature of their handicap, mentally ill and mentally deficient people are, and always will be, particularly hard to integrate into the community.'

Mrs. Braddock also urged that the implementation of local authority powers should be made mandatory:

'In scattered areas and country areas, local authorities which are not so progressive or compact as city councils or local borough councils simply will not bother to put the services into operation unless there is some form of compulsion and extended financial assistance from the Government. The Royal Commission made great play of that point.'

Other subjects of considerable discussion in this debate were the questions of research, of the care and treatment of the psychopath, and of the position of medical superintendents in mental hospitals.

There was general agreement that research was of the utmost importance. Mr. Mayhew thought that the Medical Research Council was spending 'a fabulously small amount' on research into mental illness, and pointed out that success in the research field, particularly in research into the treatment of the more serious mental illnesses, could have a 'magical' effect on the whole field. Mr. Austen Albu and Mr. Richard Fort wanted more research into the social causes and effects of mental illness—particularly follow-up studies, since, to quote Mr. Fort, 'we have been woefully inadequately informed about how many people are improved by one form of treatment or another'.

There was some disquiet about the provisions of the Bill concerning the psychopath. 'The fact is,' said Dr. Summerskill, 'that we have done little research into the problems of the psychopath.' Dr. A. D. D. Broughton was not happy about the proposal that psychopaths should be treated in general or in mental hospitals:

'I have found that they can be a very disturbing influence, tiresome to the staff, and harmful to the other patients.'

Dr. Reginald Bennett had had experience of treating psychopaths, and was prepared to say without hesitation that they were almost entirely unsuitable for hospital treatment:

'No hospital can stand more than one or two psychopaths in the whole hospital, let alone in one ward. The place becomes a bear garden. They put the other chaps up to tricks, and they are frightfully clever in finding out bright ideas for perhaps the duller members of the community or the more disturbed ones. The hospitals are going to refuse these chaps. . . . I do not think that we can really compel any hospital to admit more than it chooses to say is its maximum allowance of these appalling people.'

If the proposals of the Bill were to have any effect, special institutions would be necessary to deal with them.

The question of the position of the medical superintendent was raised by Dr. Broughton. The Bill referred throughout to 'the responsible medical officer' in a mental hospital. Was this to mean the medical superintendent, or the doctor who had immediate clinical charge of the patient? Mr. Kenneth Robinson thought that 'the medical superintendent has been abolished as far as his legal status goes', and asked for clarification; but no clarification was forthcoming (p. 170n).

The most striking fact about this debate to an outside observer is the very high level of information and discussion which it shows. There is a marked contrast with the mental health debate of February, 1954, when many members showed a great lack of even basic knowledge, muddling mental illness with mental deficiency, and admission rates with beddage. In 1959, the House showed itself alert, interested, and exceedingly well-informed. Perhaps this is as good an index as any other of the change in public opinion which had taken place in the intervening years.

A good deal of solid work was put into the Bill at the Committee stage. Ideas were tested, opinions were sought, and when the Bill returned to the Commons on May 5th, a number of amendments had been made—though, as the Minister of Health had forecast at the second reading, these were concerned with legal and administrative details, rather than with major matters of principle. There was general agreement as to principle—to an extent which is surprising when we recall the stormy controversies which this subject had evoked in Parliament in earlier generations.

It had been pointed out that, although the Bill provided provisions for the safeguard of the rights of patients compulsorily detained, by means of the new Mental Health Review Tribunals, it did not provide that patients should be informed of these rights. Many patients, and their relatives, are bewildered people who do not read Acts of Parliament, and who might have no means of knowing how and when to apply to a Tribunal—or even of the Tribunal's existence. An amendment provided that patients and their relatives should be supplied with 'such written statements of their rights and powers under this Act as may be so prescribed'.

The criterion for severe subnormality was extended. It had referred to patients 'incapable of living an independent life'; but since this was a criterion which could sensibly only apply to adults, a phrase to cover severely subnormal children was added: '. . . or will be so incapable when of an age to do so'.

The question of the four registered hospitals—that is, the private mental hospitals operating outside the Health Service—was raised. The Retreat, Cheadle Royal, St. Andrew's, Northampton, and Barnwood House all had a long tradition and a national reputation. It was therefore agreed that the Minister might make special provision for their inspection, rather than leaving them to be inspected by the local authority of the area.

A further amendment laid the duty of making application for admission to hospital or guardianship on the mental welfare officer in cases where such action was necessary. The Society of Mental Welfare Officers had pointed out that some patients might be overlooked if this was not done, and the Minister of Health agreed that the mental welfare officer should have the discretion. He or she was not to be simply 'a rubber-stamp'.

At the third reading, on May 6th, it was announced that other points made by members had been met. A circular had been sent from the Ministry of Health on May 4th to all local authorities, drawing attention to the Royal Commission's recommendation that there should be a re-orientation of the mental health services away from institutional care and towards community care. They were asked to make a review of their mental health services, and to make plans for development. In fulfilment of the resolution of January 26th, the Minister had agreed to use his powers under section 28 of the National Health Service Act to make the provision of mental health care mandatory on local authorities.

The Medical Research Council had also taken note of the views expressed in the debate, and had set up two committees for further mental health research—one on the epidemiology of mental disorder, and another on clinical psychiatry.

The Bill passed its third reading, again without a division, and then went to the House of Lords.

The Mental Health Bill in the Lords

The debate on the second reading of the Bill in the House of Lords[1] provides interesting comparisons with the past. The 1890 Act, as we have seen, was the culmination of the work of three Lord Chancellors —Selborne, Herschell and Halsbury. It was born of legal determination, and debated in the Lords by a group which still had a good deal of political power, but which knew little of the real issues at stake.

The 1959 Bill came up to the Lords from the Commons. It was introduced by the Lord Chancellor (Lord Kilmuir); but his powerful legal talents were devoted, not to legalistic definition, but to support of a Bill designed to minimize the legal elements in mental treatment. He described the Bill as 'the first fundamental revision of the English mental health laws since 1845, when the two Bills introduced by Lord Ashley,[2] later the seventh and famous Earl of Shaftesbury, created the system on which all the later additions of the last hundred years have been based'. No specific mention was made of the Act of 1890.

In 1889 and 1890, the lawyers dominated the debate. In 1959, the Lords could provide a series of experts, some hereditary peers and some life peers, to speak with knowledge and first-hand experience of varying aspects of mental health work—a psychiatrist (Lord Taylor); a social scientist (Lady Wootton); the chairman of the National Association for Mental Health (Lord Feversham); the chairman of the National Society for Mentally Handicapped Children (Lord Pakenham); and Lord Grenfell, who, in a moving speech, told the House of his own experiences as the parent of a mongol child.

After the third reading, the Lords sent the Bill back to the Commons, with a series of amendments. Many of these were concerned with exact legal definition rather than with the spirit and intention of the Act, but three proposed changes in practice. The substitution of 'remuneration' for 'fees' in the section dealing with the payment of members of Mental Health Review Tribunals was proposed, to enable the chairman or other members to be paid a permanent salary if necessary; a clause was introduced, laying on Regional Hospital Boards the duty of notifying local authorities of the availability of beds for urgent cases—this was very necessary if the hospitals were no longer to be obliged to take certain kinds of patients; and the rights of the patient in his dealings with the Mental Health Review Tribunal were clarified and extended.

[1] *Hansard*, June 4th, 1959.
[2] *Hansard* reads 'George Ashley'—probably a transcriber's error.

It is notable that the part played by the Lords in discussion and amendment of the Bill was a constructive and valuable one. Though the Upper House had lost much political power since 1890, it demonstrated, at least in this sphere, that it had still much to contribute to the national life.

The Lords' amendments were accepted by the Commons in a debate on July 24th, 1959. The Bill received the Royal Assent on July 29th.

THE MENTAL HEALTH ACT, 1959

The Act repeals all previous lunacy, mental treatment and mental deficiency legislation, and provides a single code for all types of mental disorder.

Definitions

'*Mental disorder*' is defined as 'mental illness, arrested or incomplete development of mind, psychopathic disorder, and any other disorder or disability of mind'.

'*Mental illness*' is not further defined.

'*Arrested or incomplete development of mind*' is defined under the headings 'severe subnormality' and 'subnormality'. 'Severe subnormality' is of such a nature or degree that the patient is incapable of leading an independent life, or of guarding against serious exploitation. 'Subnormality' is a condition which does not amount to severe subnormality as defined above, but which is 'susceptible to medical treatment or other special care and training of the patient'. Both must include subnormality of intelligence.

'*Psychopathic disorder*' is defined as 'a persistent disorder or disability of mind (whether or not including subnormality of intelligence) which results in abnormally aggressive or seriously irresponsible conduct . . . and requires or is susceptible to medical treatment'.

All these definitions are given in section 4 of the Act, which also contains a clause to the effect that persons are not to be regarded as suffering from a form of mental disorder 'by reason only of promiscuity or other immoral conduct'.

A *hospital* is defined as a hospital within the National Health Service, any special hospital (the former 'State Institutions' for dangerous or violent patients) and any accommodation provided by a local authority for hospital and specialist services (section 147).

A *mental nursing home* is defined as any other place for the reception of one or more patients suffering from mental disorder (section 14).

'*Medical treatment*' includes nursing care and treatment, and any kind of care and training taking place under medical supervision (section 147).

'*Local health authority*' means the council of a county or county borough, or a joint board set up for health purposes by two or more such bodies (section 147 and National Health Service Act 1946, section 19).

Administration

(i) Central. The Minister of Health was already, by the terms of the National Health Service Act, responsible for the mental health services; but the Board of Control, which had been set up in 1913 and had inherited the work of the Lunacy Commissioners, was still in existence as a quasi-independent body. The Mental Health Act dissolves the Board of Control (section 2), existing officers of the Board being transferred to the Ministry of Health. The Board's functions of inspection and review of individual cases of compulsory detention are transferred to local bodies (see below). The Minister has no overriding power of discharge of individual patients, but may refer any case to a Mental Health Review Tribunal (section 57).

(ii) Local. Local authority mental health services provided under section 28 of the National Health Service Act are to continue, and the Mental Health Act gives a statement of their powers at some length, including the provision of residential accommodation, the provision of centres for training and occupation, the appointment of mental welfare officers, the exercise of the functions of guardianship, and 'the provision of any ancillary or supplementary services' for the mentally disordered (section 6). This section simply defines in greater detail what some authorities were already doing under section 28.

Section 12 gives the local authority the power to compel children, but not adults, to attend occupation and training centres.

Mental welfare officers are given powers of entry and inspection (section 22.) They may apply to a magistrate for a warrant to search for and remove a person believed to be suffering from mental disorder (section 135). It is the duty of the mental welfare officer to make application for admission to hospital or guardianship where such action is 'necessary and proper' (section 54).

Local health authorities are designated as registration authorities for mental nursing homes (section 14). The Minister of Health may make regulations for the conduct of such homes (section 16) and may exempt the registered hospitals from local authority inspection (section 17).

Although the local health authority has the primary responsibility for mentally disordered persons through its mental health service, other local authority bodies may assume responsibility for them in suitable circumstances. Arrangements may be made for them to be housed in Part III accommodation under the National Assistance Act, 1948, which is amended for the purpose. This would bring them under the care of the welfare authority; and the children authority constituted under the Children Act, 1948, may assume responsibility for mentally disordered children (sections 8 and 9).

Mental Health Review Tribunals. These new bodies take over the 'watchdog' functions of the Board of Control. They are to review individual cases of compulsory detention at the request of patients or relatives (section 3 and section 122) or at the request of the Minister (section 57). One Tribunal is to be constituted for each Regional Hospital Board Area (section 3). The constitution of Tribunals is set out in the first schedule to the Act. They are to consist of an unspecified number of persons:

(i) Legal members, appointed by the Lord Chancellor.

(ii) Medical members, appointed by the Lord Chancellor in consultation with the Minister of Health.

(iii) Members 'having such experience in administration, such knowledge of the social services, or such other qualifications or experience as the Lord Chancellor considers suitable', also appointed by the Lord Chancellor in consultation with the Minister of Health. The chairman must be a legal member. A Tribunal sitting on any particular occasion need not call on all its members, but members present must include one or more from each of the three categories set out above, appointed by the chairman. If the chairman himself is not present, the acting chairman must be a legal member (schedule I).

Detailed rules for the regulation of Tribunal proceedings are laid down, subject to the discretion of the Lord Chancellor (section 124). Tribunals have the power to discharge patients from compulsory detention or from guardianship (section 123). Application for a hearing by a Tribunal must be made by or in respect of a patient 'by notice in writing addressed to the tribunal for the area in which the hospital or nursing home is situated' (section 122) at specific times laid down in the Act.

Admission to Hospital

(i) *Informal admission.* Hospitals are no longer obliged to take patients; but it is the duty of the Regional Hospital Board to give notice to the local health authority of where beds are available for urgent admissions (section 132).

Patients may be admitted to any hospital or mental nursing home without formalities of any kind, and without liability to detention (section 5). This clause, which is phrased negatively ('Nothing in this Act shall be construed as preventing....') replaces the previous arrangements for voluntary treatment set down in the Mental Treatment Act of 1930. Since the patient's volition is no longer required, this section can be taken to cover a large section of mental hospital patients who have no power of volition, provided that they do not positively object to treatment.

Children over the age of sixteen may be admitted for informal treatment without the consent of their parents and guardians, but only if they are capable of expressing their own wishes (section 5).

'Any hospital'. The separate designation of mental hospitals is ended. The provision of beds for mentally disordered patients becomes an administrative and clinical matter, and no longer a legal one.

(ii) *Compulsory admission.* There are three kinds of compulsory admission: admission for observation, admission for treatment, and emergency admission. These apply, like the rest of the Act, to all kinds of patients suffering from mental disorder.

An observation order is of twenty-eight days' duration. It must be made on the written recommendations of two medical practitioners who state that the patient either (*a*) is suffering from mental disorder of a nature or a degree which warrants his detention under observation for a limited period or (*b*) that he ought to be detained 'in the interests of his own health and safety, or with a view to the protection of other persons' (section 25).

A treatment order (section 26) is similarly to be signed by two general practitioners, one of whom may be on the staff of the hospital into which the patient is received,[1] and the other of whom must be appointed for the purpose by a local health authority (section 28). The duration of a treatment order is for periods of one year, one year, one year, and then two years at a time (section 43). The grounds for recommendation of admission by treatment are three-fold—the conditions are not alternative, like those for admission by observation, but must all be fulfilled:

(*a*) The patient must be suffering from mental illness or severe subnormality; or from subnormality or psychopathic disorder if he is under the age of twenty-one.

(*b*) He must suffer from this disorder to an extent which, in the minds of the recommending doctors, warrants detention in hospital for medical treatment under this section; *and* his detention must be necessary in the interests of his own health and safety, or for the protection of other persons.

An emergency order (section 29) lasts only for three days. The application must be made by a mental welfare officer or a relative of the patient, and backed by one medical recommendation. No grounds for this recommendation are laid down, but the patient must be discharged after three days unless a further medical recommendation has been given, satisfying the conditions of section 28 (i.e. for a treatment order).

These clauses are a development from existing practice, the main change being the abolition of a magistrate's order in admission for treatment.

Care and Treatment in Hospital

The Minister may provide pocket money for patients who would otherwise be 'without resources to meet personal expenses' (section 133).

[1] But not in the case of a private patient, or of admission to a mental nursing home, i.e. the hospital doctor can only give such a recommendation where his own financial interest is not involved.

Patients are not to be ill-treated or wilfully neglected by the managers or staff of hospitals or mental nursing homes (sections 126).

Mentally ill and severely subnormal women are protected against unlawful sexual intercourse (section 127).

No restrictions are placed on the correspondence of patients informally admitted (section 134). The correspondence of patients liable to compulsory detention may be supervised by the 'responsible medical officer' in two ways: he may keep a letter written by a patient from the post if it is offensive or defamatory, or if it is likely to prejudice the interests of the patient; or if the addressee in a particular case has requested that letters should not be forwarded. Letters addressed to certain people, including the Minister of Health, any Member of Parliament, and a member of a Mental Health Review Tribunal at a time when the patient's case is due for review, must be forwarded in all cases, and are not within the discretion of the 'responsible medical officer' (section 36). Letters written to a patient are also subject to supervision: the 'responsible medical officer' may withhold a letter if he feels that its delivery might interfere with the patient's treatment, or cause him unnecessary distress (section 36).

Visitation. Any medical practitioner appointed by the patient or a relative may visit and examine the patient in private, for the purpose of advising whether an application should be made to a Mental Health Review Tribunal; or of advising the nearest relative on the question of the patient's suitability for discharge by the exercise of his special rights (see below under 'Discharge'). The Regional Hospital Board or the registration authority may send visitors, medical or lay, to have private interviews with patients in mental nursing homes (section 37).

Leave of Absence. The 'responsible medical officer' may grant any patient leave of absence for up to six months, making any conditions which he considers necessary for the patient's custody and welfare, 'in the interests of the patient or for the protection of other persons'.

If a patient liable to be detained is absent without leave, he may be taken into custody and returned to the hospital within a specified period by any mental welfare officer, any constable, any member of the hospital's staff, or any other person authorized in writing by the managers of the hospital or the local health authority. The specified period is six months in the case of a psychopathic or subnormal patient between the ages of twenty-one and twenty-five who is liable to detention on a treatment or guardianship order; and twenty-eight days in all other cases (section 40).

Discharge

A patient is discharged when the order requiring his detention lapses; or by the 'responsible medical officer' or the managers of the hospital or mental nursing home (section 47) or by a Mental Health Review Tribunal after application and hearing (section 123); or, if, in the case of a subnormal or psychopathic patient, he was detained on a treatment order before he was twenty-one, and has now reached the age of twenty-five; or any patient on a treatment order can be discharged at seventy-two hours' notice by his nearest relative, provided that the 'responsible medical officer' does not certify that he would be 'likely to act in a manner dangerous to other persons or himself' (section 48). 'Nearest relative' is defined in some detail in section 49.

Guardianship

The concept of guardianship which had its origin in the Mental Deficiency Acts may now be applied to all types of patients suffering from mental disorder. An application for guardianship may be made on the grounds that:

(a) the patient is suffering from mental illness or severe subnormality; or that he is under the age of twenty-one, and suffering from psychopathic disorder or subnormality;

(b) that the disorder is of such a nature or degree as to warrant a guardianship order;

(c) that the guardianship order is necessary in the interests of the patient, or for the protection of other persons.

The guardian appointed may be an individual (possibly the individual making the application) or a local health authority (section 33). A guardianship order is of the same duration, and, subject to relevant modifications, of the same type and conditions as a treatment order.

Patients Concerned in Criminal Proceedings

This part of the Act gives Courts of Assize, Quarter Sessions, and magistrates' courts power to order admission to a specified hospital or guardianship for patients of all ages suffering from mental disorder of any kind (section 60). The recommendation of two medical practitioners is required, and one of these must be a psychiatrist approved by a local health authority (section 62). Courts of Assize and Quarter Sessions may place special restrictions on the discharge of such patients (section 65). Power to grant leave of absence, to transfer the patient to another hospital, or to cancel any restrictions placed on his discharge, is reserved to the Home Secretary (sections 65 and 66). Limitations are placed on the appeal of such patients to Mental Health Review Tribunals (section 63). The normal right of the nearest relative to discharge does not apply to them (section 63).

Prisoners detained 'during Her Majesty's pleasure' may be detained in hospital by warrant from the Home Secretary (section 71).

Prisoners already in custody or serving a sentence of imprisonment may be transferred to hospital or to guardianship by warrant from the Home Secretary (sections 72 and 73).

An order for a prisoner to be detained in hospital ceases to have effect at the time when his sentence of imprisonment would have expired; and a prisoner who recovers from his mental illness before the expiry of his sentence may be returned to prison to serve the remainder (sections 78 and 76).

The provisions of this part of the Act also apply to children and young persons in connection with Borstals or approved schools.

Management of Patients' Property and Affairs

This part of the Act confirms the existing system for safeguarding a patients' financial interests through the offices of the Court of Protection. It codifies and extends the law relating to the management of property for or on behalf of a person suffering from mental disorder (sections 100-19).

Members of Parliament

A section which gave rise to some comment in the Press was that relating to members of the House of Commons. This lays down special procedures for ascertaining the mental condition of a member of the House of Commons through notification to the Speaker; and provides that, if the member is compulsorily detained by reason of mental disorder for more than six months, his seat in the House shall become vacant. This does not extend to members of the House of Lords (section 137).

.   .   .   .   .

This is a brief summary of the main provisions of a long and complex Act, which, at the time of writing, has not yet come into operation. It is difficult therefore to comment at length on its terms, since so much remains to be worked out in practice, and the discretion allowed to the Minister of Health and the Lord Chancellor for making regulations is so great. In particular, this discretion applies to the Minister's promise to make certain powers of local authorities mandatory; to the constitution and practice of Mental Health Review Tribunals; and to the question of how and by what means patients are made aware of their rights under the Act.

On the eve of the Act's coming into operation, some mental welfare officers are nervous of their new powers and responsibilities; and some are worried lest the 'battle of wits' for hospital beds should grow more acute when the onus of finding a bed rests with the remote Regional Hospital Board rather than with the individual hospital. The recommendations of the Younghusband Committee on local authority conditions of service and training for health and welfare workers have not yet come into effect, so that the mental welfare officer is at present in some doubt about his future sphere of action, and his future relations with the hospital service; but the publication of the Younghusband Report and the passing of the Mental Health Act have done much to arouse the interest and intelligence of mental welfare workers—and indeed of local health authorities as a whole.

Criticism of the clauses relating to the psychopath has in particular been directed against the concept that the psychopath should not be liable to compulsory detention after the age twenty-five; and against the requirement that he can only be detained between the ages of twenty-one and twenty-five if the original order was made before his twenty-first birthday. 'Psychopathic disorder' is defined as 'a persistent disorder or disability of mind . . . which results in abnormally aggressive or seriously irresponsible conduct and which requires or is susceptible to medical treatment'. Thus a patient may be *clinically* described as a psychopath, but not *legally* a psychopath, if suitable care, treatment or training is not in existence. As yet, there is no clear agreement between psychiatrists in this country on the question of active and successful treatment for psychopaths; and the intention of the Act seems to preclude a simple detention while the patient's belated emotional development takes place. If hospitals have the right to accept or refuse patients, what hospitals will take the psychopath, often the greatest trouble-maker in the mental hospital population? Will special hospitals be built for them? How soon—and how will staff be recruited?

It should be noted that the definition of subnormality and severe subnormality differs from the definitions of feeble-mindedness and idiocy or imbecility previously in use, because it includes low intelligence. As we have seen, previous practice was to regard mental deficiency as a failure of social adjustment rather than a failure of educational ability. As a result, those 'moral defectives' previously dealt with under the Mental Deficiency Acts will now be dealt with as psychopaths.

The question of the 'responsible medical officer' has not yet been settled. The Act merely defines him as 'the medical practitioner in charge of the treatment of the patient'; but who is 'in charge'? The Registrar or senior House Medical Officer who actually carries out treatment? The consultant who is responsible for supervising his work? Or the medical superintendent? This question has not yet been settled, and there may be local variations in practice unless the Minister settles the question by regulation.

The Act, like many legal documents, spends a good deal of space over minute legal issues, while major social and medical issues are disposed of in a few words. The most striking clause in the whole document is that short and unobtrusive section 5, which relates to informal admission to hospital, and does not define the kind of hospital to which it applies. This clause will mean a much greater freedom for many mental patients, and may be as instrumental in bringing about a new attitude to mental disorder as the Mental Treatment Act of 1930 was in its own day, with its regulations as to voluntary patients.

The provisions for guardianship may mean a new step forward. Again, it remains to be seen how these provisions will operate in practice; but it may be possible for many patients other than mental defectives to be dealt with in this way, particularly old people in local authority guardianship—possibly in half-way houses or other accommodation of this type.

The intention of the Act is to free all but a few patients from compulsory detention. It walks the tight-rope between the freedom of the individual and the liberty of the subject carefully: a patient may be detained 'in the interests of his own health and safety, or with a view to the protection of other persons'; but this will only be done as a last resort, after efforts to get him to enter hospital voluntarily have failed.

The Act codifies, simplifies, and amends the previous Law on the subject. Where it amends, it initiates boldly and clearly in harmony with modern clinical and social views of mental disorder. In providing a single code for all forms of mental disorder, in threading a way through the complexity of the old lunacy and mental treatment and mental deficiency laws, it has taken the best of the old system, and left scope for future development.

EPILOGUE

THIS survey set out to chart the changing response of English society to a series of questions—What is mental disorder? What forms of care should the community provide? Who should be responsible for administering them? How far is it necessary to compel patients to receive treatment against their will? How can this be done without infringing the essential liberty of the subject? A comparison of today's answers with those of 1845 shows how far we have moved in theory and practice in a little over a hundred years.

The answers in 1845 would have run something like this: insanity is an affliction of the mind. It is quite different from physical illness, and quite unlike normal behaviour. It is generally caused by poor heredity, or by drink, or possibly by starvation. Insane people should be sent to asylums, and most of them will have to stay there for life. Special authorities should be set up for the purpose of running asylums, under a strong central control. Patients have to be treated under compulsion, and they must be locked in, in case they try to escape. The only way in which they can be detained without infringing the liberty of the subject is to delay certification until the patient is obviously, and perhaps incurably, abnormal. Early treatment might mean wrongful detention in some cases, and our first duty is to protect the sane.

In 1959, the response is very different. In an extremely simplified form, it might be expressed thus: mental disorder is a loose general term covering a number of conditions about which we still have much to learn. There is a close relationship to physical disorder. There is no hard and fast line between 'normal' and 'abnormal', but rather a series of gradations between the well-adjusted at one end of the scale, and those who are unable to adjust to the demands of society at the other.

The community should provide a wide range of forms of care, from complete hospital treatment to domiciliary visiting. The mental hospital or mental deficiency hospital is only one tool in the hands of the psychiatrist and his colleagues, and many patients need never enter hospital at all. Those who do have a good chance of returning home within three to six months. Even if they relapse, it is better for them to have short periods of hospital treatment than to spend their whole lives in an institution.

The best form of administration is one which considers the needs of individuals, rather than dividing them into arbitrary categories for administrative convenience. There is no need for all mental patients to be dealt with by a single organization. A number of different health and welfare services may be used in varying circumstances.

Compulsion is rarely necessary—only when a patient is endangering his own safety or that of other people. The vast majority of patients can be admitted freely, and allowed to leave at their own request. When mental hospitals have open doors, and patients are given as much freedom as they can reasonably deal with, there is less incentive to leave against the advice of the psychiatrist.

In this situation, the question of infringing the liberty of the subject seldom arises. In any case, in a nationalized health service, no-one gains an advantage from detaining a patient: it is in everybody's interest to restore him to his family as quickly as possible; but if the question of wrongful detention should be raised, a local tribunal will provide a speedier and more effective hearing than an appeal to a distant central authority.

In some ways, we have reversed the administrative trends of 1845. Then the problem was to separate out the 'insane' from the poor and the sick and the criminal, to provide a special service for them, and to centralize. Now the pendulum swings back: the mentally disordered are dispersed again to the care of a number of services—though in a very different social setting. Administrative centralization reached its peak in the National Health Service, and we have begun a degree of decentralization through local authorities and local tribunals.

Administrative answers depend on circumstances. The workers have changed: in place of the few 'asylum doctors' and 'attendants', we have a whole range of specialists—psychiatrists, psychologists, social workers, nurses and others—each group with a body of knowledge and techniques of its own. The patients have changed—for only a very small proportion of the people who come within the scope of the mental health services today bear any obvious relation to the unhappy 'lunatics' of 1845. Many have milder forms of mental disorder which would not have been recognized then. Others are treated at an earlier stage, and our society does not let them reach the demented and degraded depths to which a human being could sink in the mid-nineteenth century. The standard of living is much higher, and the family has recourse to many forms of social aid, so that discharge does not mean, as it so often did a century ago, a return to conditions of wretchedness and near-starvation. Public opinion has changed; for in the last few years, television, radio and press have been enlisted in the campaign to abolish fear and prejudice, the last remnants of the witch-hunt. The administrative setting has changed. Within the scope of the welfare state, there is room for flexibility in methods of care; within a central framework, there is room for decentralization, for local initiative and experiment.

So the answers we give to the fundamental questions about mental disorder change, and perhaps will change again. For there is nothing final about the solutions of 1959. Administrative principles alter in response to circumstances. Only the ethical principle remains constant.

Appendix One

STATISTICS OF MENTAL DISORDER

I. TOTAL NUMBER OF KNOWN PERSONS OF UNSOUND MIND, 1859–1909

Jan. 1	Known persons of unsound mind (thousands)	Rate of increase	Estimated total pop. of England and Wales (millions)	Percentage of known persons of unsound mind in total population
1859	31·4	—	19·6	·160
1864	38·7	+7·3	20·0	·188
1869	46·7	+8·0	21·5	·217
1874	54·3	+7·6	23·0	·236
1879	61·6	+7·3	25·2	·244
1884	69·9	+8·3	25·2	·277
1889	75·6	+5·7	28·4	·266
1894	83·0	+7·4	29·8	·279
1899	95·6	+12·6	31·6	·303
1904	117·2	+21·6	33·6	·349
1909	128·2	+11·0	35·0	·366

Figures for known persons of unsound mind 1859–99 are taken from the 54th Report of the Lunacy Commissioners, 1900, Appendix A. Figures for total population estimated from decennial Census returns. These figures are not accurate in detail, but merely indicate a general trend.

'Known persons of unsound mind' includes both 'lunatics' and 'idiots', and all patients whether in public asylums, private hospitals, private nursing homes or single care; but not those in workhouses, or prisons, for whom no figures appear to have been kept. The rising percentage probably indicates not a rise in the proportion of insane persons, but an increasing awareness of what was previously at least in part a submerged social problem; the diligence of the Lunacy Commissioners in identifying and listing patients in small private nursing homes and single care; and the increasing provision in public asylums (see Table 3). In particular, the steep rise shown in the figures for 1899 and 1904 is

207

related to new accommodation built after the 1890 Act, when fewer patients were sent to workhouses.

2. TOTAL NUMBER OF PERSONS RECEIVING INSTITUTIONAL TREATMENT FOR MENTAL ILLNESS, 1904–54

Jan. 1	In-patients (thousands)	Rate of increase	Estimated total pop. of England and Wales (millions)	% of in-patients
1914	138·1	+9·3	36·6	·377
1919	116·7	−21·4	37·7	·309
1924	130·3	+13·6	38·4	·339
1929	141·1	+10·8	39·6	·356
1934	150·3	+9·2	40·5	·371
1939⎫ 1944⎭	no figures available			
1949	144·7	−5·6	43·3	·334
1954	151·4	+6·7	44·0	·344

Figures for in-patients taken from Annual Reports of the Board of Control. These include patients in State Institutions, mental nursing homes and general hospitals, as well as mental hospitals. Figures for total population estimated from Census returns. The total percentage of persons receiving in-patient treatment was higher in 1914 than it has ever been since. This is due to the sharp drop in accommodation and treatment facilities resulting from two World Wars, the transfer of mental defectives to mental deficiency hospitals as accommodation became available; but mainly to the increasing provision of out-patient treatment through clinics and (latterly) local authority care. No national figures for out-patients are available.

3. MENTAL DEFECTIVES UNDER STATUTORY FORMS OF CARE, 1947–57

Dec. 31	Patients in in institutions	Under guardianship or notified	Under statutory supervision	Total
1947	54,229	5,373	43,719	103,321
1948	54,887	5,724	44,787	105,398
1949	56,506	4,558	47,158	108,222
1950	56,726	4,095	48,295	109,116
1951	57,661	3,850	50,049	111,560
1952	59,006	3,690	56,140	118,836
1953	60,065	3,446	55,452	118,963
1954	60,868	3,303	57,734	121,905
1955	61,439	3,135	59,594	124,168
1956	60,927	3,084	60,467	124,478
1957	60,919	2,939	60,388	124,246

STATISTICS OF MENTAL DISORDER

Figures taken in all cases from the Annual Reports of the Ministry of Health. 'Patients in institutions' includes those in hospitals vested in the Minister of Health, Rampton and Moss Side institutions, certified institutions and approved homes, and patients on licence. They show an increase in institutional care and in statutory supervision, and a considerable decrease in guardianship and notification. The decrease is probably due to a greater use of voluntary supervision, for which no figures are available. The increase in total numbers ascertained, though marked, similarly does not take account of those cases where no statutory action was taken.

The Board of Control gave no clear figures for the number of mental defectives before 1947.

Appendix Two

THE SIZE OF MENTAL HOSPITALS
(COUNTY ASYLUMS)

Jan. 1	No. of county county borough and city asylums	Total patients in public asylums	Average number of patients per asylum
1827	9	1,046	116
1850	24	7,140	297
1860	41	15,845	386
1870	50	27,109	542
1880	61	40,088	657
1890	66	52,937	802
1900	77	74,004	961
1910	91	97,580	1,072
1920	94	93,648 (104,298)	996 (1,109)
1930	98	119,659	1,221

Figures for number of asylums and total patients in asylums taken from Annual Reports of the Lunacy Commissioners before 1913, Board of Control after 1913. Figures in parentheses for 1920 are those for the total numbers of beds available, as distinct from the total number of beds occupied. Many beds had then recently been freed from use as emergency beds for war cases, and the normal flow of civilian cases had not yet been resumed. No figures are available for 1940, as no reports were issued during the war period. Figures for the period since the inception of the National Health Service would be misleading, since a number of mental patients are now accommodated in psychiatric wards or units attached to general hospitals. The statistics for the average number of patients per asylum indicate strikingly the rise in the size of asylums which was partly responsible for the loss of human relationships in asylum administration and the common policy in this respect, which was to add to the size of existing asylums rather than building new ones, from motives of economy.

Appendix Three

THE ROYAL COMMISSION ON
MENTAL ILLNESS AND
MENTAL DEFICIENCY, 1954–7

THE evidence presented to the Commission by the Ministry of Health and the Board of Control is of particular interest, since it represented the most highly-informed and official view of the shape which future legislation should take. Though the Board of Control was still in law an independent body, it had come into close administrative liaison with the Ministry since 1948. A joint memorandum was submitted, and oral evidence was given by Mr. (now Sir Frederick) Armer, and the Hon. W. S. Maclay, with other members of the Board of Control.[1] Mr. Armer was then Chairman of the Board of Control, and a permanent official of the Ministry of Health. Dr. Maclay was Senior Medical Commissioner of the Board.

The recommendations made to the Royal Commission in the written memorandum included the abolition of all formalities in voluntary admission to mental hospital; the simplification of certification procedure; the extension of arrangements, without limitation of time, for absence on leave or trial, and boarding out; the formulation of new classifications for types of mental defect; the extension of local authority powers and duties in respect of the provision of residential accommodation; and the diminution or abolition of the special functions of the Board of Control as Mental Health became absorbed into the general administrative pattern of the Health Services.

Appendix A to the memorandum consisted of a useful summary of admission procedure then in existence. It is notable that procedures were so complicated that even a summary required a chart some fifteen inches square, printed in very small print. Other appendices gave statistical information which showed that, though the total number of patients resident in mental hospitals was little higher in 1952 than in 1929, the number of admissions and discharges had practically

---

[1] Minutes of Evidence, 1st day, May 4th, 1954.

tripled.[1] In the same period, the number of mental defectives under care had more than doubled. Appendix E contained a brief note on the volume of documentary work undertaken by the Board of Control. Over 2,000 documents were scrutinized weekly by the Commissioner-on-duty under legal requirement, and a further 2,000 or more were scrutinized by other officials of the Board.[2] If the Board's recommendations concerning informal admission were adopted, much of this work would disappear. Other documents could be scrutinized locally rather than being dealt with at central Government level. It was clear that the scrutinization of over 4,000 documents concerning individual patients every week was administratively unworkable.

Mr. Armer stated in evidence that the Ministry and the Board considered that there was no shortage of beds for the mentally ill, with two important qualifications: many of the beds were not in suitable accommodation—'a great deal of it is very bad'—and many of the beds were wrongly used, being filled with a number of stabilized chronic patients and mildly senile patients who did not require the full resources of a hospital, and should be cared for in the community. In mental deficiency, the picture was rather different, and the existing accommodation was inadequate; but community care was rapidly increasing, particularly for high-grade defectives. In both cases, the development of adequate community care would greatly reduce the demand for hospital beds.

Dr. Maclay, in giving evidence on the administrative procedure of voluntary admission and discharge, told a story which illustrated vividly the changing attitudes to the mental hospital

'... when I was at the Bethlem Hospital once, there was a patient struggling at the front door with two male nurses, and the Superintendent turned to me and said "You may think that is a patient being restrained against his will, but it is a voluntary patient being discharged".'

A question to which the Commission gave much attention was the matter of the stigma involved in certification of mental patients. Sir Russell Brain asked, 'What is the factor to which the stigma attaches?' The members of the Board of Control felt that it lay in the magistrate's order. 'Our view,' stated Mr. Armer, 'is that you should avoid procedure before a magistrate as much as you can.' On the third day of the enquiry, Mr. Hudd, secretary of the Society of Chief Administrative Mental Health Officers, in an exchange with Mr. (now Sir Harry) Hylton-Foster, elaborated this point

'(Mr. Hylton-Foster) You say that the intervention of the magistrate adds to the stigma, and that presumably means in the mind of the patient, and in the

[1] Patients resident 1929: 137,744.
　　　　　　　　1952: 148,122.
　　Discharges 1929: 10,494.
　　　　　　　1952: 33,756.
[2] i.e. notices of admission, death or discharge and medical certificates required under the Lunacy and Mental Treatment and the Mental Deficiency Acts.

mind of the patient's relatives. I am not indicating any views, but can you say why?

—If I may say so, it is the legal formalities. The more people who are brought into the picture, the worse the position becomes for the patient.

—It is, as it were, the heaviness of the procedure?

—That is right, Sir.'

Sir Cecil Oakes felt that the stigma lay, not in the procedure, but in the institution, as far as ex-patients and their relatives were concerned.

'They do not know anything about the certificate, they do not understand it. They do not know their brother is certified, they do not know their mother is certified; it is simply having to go to the institution.'

Witnesses and members of the Commission were quick to point out that this did not seem to operate in the case of voluntary patients, who entered mental hospital of their own accord. Dr. T. P. Rees felt that the real stigma lay in the fact of compulsion against the patient's will. Voluntary patients in mental hospitals tended to feel 'superior'.

Dr. Yellowlees, asked for his personal opinion on the second day, put another point of view. He felt that judicial intervention was 'definitely and greatly in the interests of the patient' and was also a safeguard to the doctor who provided the certificate. 'The public thinks that it is due to the doctor's wishes, prejudices and theories that people are confined in mental hospital.'

While there was much disagreement concerning which factor in certification was most responsible for the stigma, all witnesses were agreed that a sigma did exist; and that the most practicable remedy was to avoid certification and its corollary, compulsion, wherever possible.

There was a good deal of discussion on the question of the certification of mental defectives. The National Council for Civil Liberties, a voluntary society established in 1934, had published in 1951 a pamphlet entitled *50,000 outside the Law* which dealt with 200 cases in which wrongful certification was alleged. This pamphlet alleged that wrongful certification and wrongful detention still existed on a wide scale, that the Law was being administered 'in a far from humane manner', and that use of patient labour in institutions, and the practice of releasing defectives on licence to private employers, created a vested interest in continuing certification so that useful workers could be exploited by low wage-scales.

Although the pamphlet was couched in alarmist language, the evidence given before the Royal Commission by the National Council for Civil Liberties was generally restrained and helpful. It had a value in directing the Commission's attention to individual cases in a sphere where the consideration of the individual could only too easily be lost in a welter of generalizations about administrative and legal procedure. The National Council suggested that voluntary admission to hospital should be introduced for mental defectives as for mental patients with the difference that the volition would be that of the parent or guardian, not the patient. They recommended that detention of high-grade non-delinquent defectives 'should be explicitly rejected because of its cruelty, the uncertainty of its basis, and the extent to which it can be used to satisfy irrational prejudices and conceptions'; and that young defectives of this kind might well be dealt with under the Children and Young Persons' legislation. 'The fact that the individual is an orphan or has unsatisfactory parents or home conditions should be no grounds for detention' (Day 22).

Another point of much discussion was the question of the psychopath. Mr. Armer thought (Day 1) that 'a mentally defective person might be someone of normal intelligence who has defects of character, but those defects of character must have appeared . . . before the age of eighteen . . . . I think it is quite clear that many psychopaths could be dealt with as feeble-minded'.

This definition involved construing 'mind' to include affect as well as intelligence, and was contested by other witnesses.[1] The British Medical Association (Day 26) gave a clear outline of the symptoms of psychopathy

'Their persistent anti-social method of conduct may include inefficiency and lack of interest in any form of occupation; pathological lying, swindling and slandering; alcoholism and drug addiction; sexual offences and violent actions with little motivation and an entire absence of self-restraint which may go as far as homicide. Punishment or the threat of punishment influences their behaviour only momentarily, and its more lasting effect, if any, is to intensify their vindictiveness. . . .')[2]

—and believed that only a certain proportion of psychopaths could be absorbed into the populations of mental hospitals. Separate institutions were necessary for the reception of some patients, including those sent from the Courts under the Criminal Justice Act, 1948. Since the behaviour of the psychopath was so highly anti-social, there was a case for some procedure whereby they could be brought under care by compulsion before they committed acts which brought them into conflict with the criminal law; but 'safeguards of an exceptional nature should be provided', since it was obviously undesirable that any and every form of anti-social behaviour should be potential grounds for certification on this score. The National Association for Mental Health (Day 28) thought that such procedure should only be employed in connection with the aggressive psychopath. The Society of Chief Administrative Mental Health Officers (Day 3) wanted them kept out of mental hospitals at all costs. 'You are going to turn the mental hospitals into some sort of prison.'

The Society also took up the question of the powers and duties of local authorities. They believed that the powers which devolved from section 28 of the National Health Service Act were so vaguely phrased that many local

[1] See evidence of the British Psychological Society. Day 17, p. 607.
[2] This statement was actually drafted by the Royal Medico-Psychological Association and adopted almost *in toto* by the B.M.A.

authorities were administering them, particularly with regard to mental defectives, 'in a very half-hearted way'. Clearer definition was necessary especially where their powers to provide residential accommodation were concerned. 'Throughout the whole of the country, there is no real uniformity either in practice or general administration as regards the mental health work of local authorities.' The Royal Medico-Psychological Association concurred (Day 8) and pointed out that the tripartite system of administration in the health service was hampering the development of local authority work.

The Society of Mental Welfare Officers brought up the major issue of whether it was wise, in framing new legislation, to consider mental illness and mental deficiency together.

'We consider these to be separate problems. The public often shows little appreciation of the difference between mental illness and mental deficiency, and in our opinion, the suggestion of a combined Act covering these subjects is unwise, tending to confuse the issue at a time when great efforts are being made to educate the public in matters appertaining to Mental Health' (Day 5). This matter was not taken up in oral evidence.

THE REPORT OF THE ROYAL COMMISSION, 1957

(i) Basic Definitions

The Royal Commission decided to use the term 'mental disorder' as a generic phrase to cover all forms of mental ill-health, mental illness, mental deficiency, and the psychopathic states. They recognized that this might initially lead to some difficulty since 'mental disorder' was usually used as a synonym for mental illness; but after considering and rejecting such alternatives as 'mental abnormality' and 'mental unfitness', they concluded, 'We do not consider that using the term "mental disorder" in this comprehensive sense should lead to misunderstanding or confusion, and we prefer it to any alternative that we have been able to think of.'

It was recommended that, within this main category, three main groups of patients should be recognized for legal and administrative purposes. (That is, these were not clinical definitions. Legal definitions in this field are concerned with social classification, not with medical diagnosis and treatment.)

(a) Mentally ill patients. This group included those suffering from the mental infirmity of old age. The phrase 'person of unsound mind' would no longer be used.

(b) Psychopathic patients. The term 'psychopathic personality' was used to include all types of aggressive or inadequate behaviour which did not render the patient severely subnormal, and which was 'recognized medically as a pathological condition'.

(c) Severely subnormal patients. 'When the general personality is so severely subnormal that the patient is incapable of leading an independent life.' This would include idiots, imbeciles, and some feeble-minded patients, but not all.

(ii) Administration

Generally, the Commission considered it essential that the mental health services should remain integrated with the general health and welfare services, and that the degree of integration should be increased in the future. The health and welfare services had been reorganized since 1948 on a functional basis—the main criterion for administrative classification being not 'What kind of person is this?' but 'What kind of need has this person?' Where the needs of a mentally disordered person could be dealt with through the general social services, this was preferable to designating a special service for them, which set them apart.

The abolition of the Board of Control was a recommendation which reflected this attitude. It was considered that the existence of a separate inspectorate nominally outside the Ministry of Health was 'neither necessary nor desirable'. The Ministry could arrange regular inspections of hospitals, if these were thought necessary, by qualified officers from its own staff. The scrutinization of documents, where it continued to be necessary, should be carried out by the medical, clerical and welfare personnel concerned in completing them. Such documents should be kept, and should be available to officers of the Ministry of Health, members of Mental Health Review Tribunals, and other officials upon request.

The Board of Control was already working in very close liaison with the Ministry of Health, and was actually situated in the Ministry of Health building in London. Its abolition, therefore, would involve merely the administrative transfer of its staff to the Ministry staff, and a greater freedom of action once the routine work of annual visits to hospitals and regular scrutinization of documents had ended.

The Board's work of investigating individual cases would be taken over by the new Mental Health Review Tribunals, which were recommended for each Regional Hospital Board area. These tribunals should have the power to review cases of compulsory detention on specific occasions, such as when the patient was first admitted, or when his certificate was due for renewal. They should be composed of medical and non-medical members selected from a panel of suitable persons in each region. It was felt that local investigation would be more valuable than that of a remote central body; and that a medical and lay panel would be preferable to a panel of magistrates, since it was no longer necessary to stress the legal element in mental disorder. The non medical part of the panel might be composed of some people with legal knowledge, some with administrative experience, and some with knowledge and experience of the social services. No member should be selected to serve on a panel hearing a case with which he had a direct connection through a hospital or local authority. It should be possible for patients or relatives to appeal from the decision of the tribunal to the High Courts on technical points of law only.

It was not easy to forecast the amount of work which would face the Mental Health Review Tribunals. The Commission was inclined to think that it would not be very great but they hoped that a fairly large number of people would be appointed to regional panels, since they felt that continued hearing of appeals of this sort, many of which had to be rejected, blunted the perceptions. This was one argument against a central review—'it is only too easy for anyone who is frequently considering applications which have to be refused to become less alert to recognize the rarer cases where the application should be allowed'.

At local level, it was important to distinguish between the functions of the local authority and those of the hospital, so that each would recognize the full responsibilities placed upon it. The general division of functions should be on the basis of whether the patient was in need of medical and/or nursing treatment. 'No patient should be retained as a hospital in-patient when he has reached the stage where he could return home if he had a reasonably good home to go to. At that stage, the provision of residential care becomes the responsibility of the local authority.'

The local authority should make arrangements for preventive work; and for the provision of all types of community care, including residential care—training and occupation centres for mental defectives, both children and adults, convalescent centres for patients after hospitalization, homes for psychopaths, homes for old people. 'Social help and advice should be available to all patients and to their relatives.'

There should be close co-operation between the health and education authorities where the question of training and education for severely sub-normal children was concerned. Local education authorities should have as wide a range of services for children of low ability as they felt able to provide. Similarly, there should be liaison with the children's department concerning sub-normal (but not severely subnormal) children unable to live in their own homes, who should be treated as much like other deprived children as possible; and with the welfare department concerning the aged and infirm. In the last case, where there was known to be much practical difficulty due to the general unwillingness of welfare services to deal with psychogeriatric cases, it was recommended that the Minister of Health should make a direction to the effect that the provision of residential accommodation for mentally infirm old people was a positive duty, binding on local authorities. These points were all extensions of the general principle of functionalism, and suggested a means whereby many of the mentally disordered might gradually be absorbed into the general social services.

As far as severely subnormal children were concerned, the Commission did not feel able to recommend, as some witnesses had asked, that all training and occupation of defectives carried out by the local authority should be transferred from the health department to the education department. While recognizing the shock and unhappiness of the parent who was told 'Your child is ineducable', they insisted that the form of words, not the administrative transfer, was wrong. It should be possible to recommend a child for 'special training' without creating this special form of stigma.

There should be no special designation of hospitals for one type of patient only. 'The arrangements should be capable of adaptation as medical developments may require, and there should be no legal barrier preventing the admission of any patient to any hospital which provides the sort of treatment which he is thought to need.' This recommendation was designed to bring mental hospitals in line with other types of hospital, and to do away with unnecessary legalism. It would also make it easier to treat mixed forms of mental ill-health. A somewhat retarded mental patient might benefit from a special course run at a mental deficiency institution, or a mental defective might develop a neurosis which required treatment in mental hospital. Although rigid classification has never been fully achieved—there are still mental defectives in mental hospitals, who were first admitted before mental deficiency accommodation became available—the tendency towards clear-cut grading had been growing. Again, this recommendation was on functional lines—the need was to be considered rather than the category. The placing of a psychopath would depend on the individual circumstances of the case, and on the availability or otherwise of places in special institutions.

(iii) Admission and Discharge

It was recommended that patients should be admitted to mental hospitals and mental deficiency institutions without formalities of any kind where possible, and that 'the assumption that compulsory powers must be used unless the patient can express a positive desire for treatment' should be replaced by 'the offer of care, without deprivation of liberty, to all who need it, and are not unwilling to receive it'. The difference is that between being required to contract in, and having the opportunity to contract out. It meant that a fairly large class of patients who were not capable of expressing volition specifically, but who equally had no specific objection to treatment, could be dealt with on an informal basis, where the existing law required their certification or 'temporary' admission. The use of compulsory powers was to become an exception, not a regular practice. 'Compulsory powers should then be used only when they are positively necessary to override the wishes of the patient or his relatives for the patient's own welfare or for the protection of others.'

For patients who could express volition, it meant the end of the present formalities—signing a form requesting treatment before admission, and giving seventy-two hours' notice of intention to discharge themselves. Informal admission carried the corollary of informal discharge.

In mental deficiency institutions, this implied a totally new principle, since the Mental Deficiency Acts provided only for admission under compulsion, and discharge at the instance of the statutory authorities. The initiative here would rest with the parents or guardian of the patient.

The Commission recognized that there might be some administrative difficulties in the wide extension of arrangements for informal admission which was envisaged. Hospital authorities might have difficulty in making adequate arrangements with relatives and mental health departments if patients could discharge themselves without notice, but the Commission pointed out that there were already informally-admitted mental patients in general hospitals, in neurosis units, and in 'de-designated' wards[1] of mental hospitals. The Commission felt that the system was workable, and that mental hospital staffs could deal with the problems involved. A second argument against informal admission was that the patient, in signing a form requesting admission, was made aware of the fact that it was necessary for him to accept the rules of the hospital, including possible restrictions on his freedom of movement, but it was felt that the patient should be expected to accept such rules and restrictions as a condition of joining the hospital community. If he objected to doing so, he could leave the hospital.

A further question was that of procedure where the patient was willing to receive further treatment and his doctor considered further treatment necessary, but the patient's relatives pressed for discharge. It was recommended that, if the patient was over the age of sixteen, he should be asked to sign a statement saying that he wished to stay in the hospital, and realized that he was free to leave the hospital when he wished. If the patient was under the age of sixteen, then the relatives' wishes would have to be respected, and the patient discharged.

'There can be no question of a barring certificate, even on the grounds of danger to the patient or to others, in relation to patients admitted informally, when the hospital has no authority to detain.'

By contrast with the sections on informal admission, those on compulsion occupy a considerable part of the report, though it was hoped that they would refer to an increasingly dwindling number of patients. Chapter 6 of the Report begins with a consideration of the philosophical background of compulsion.

'There is a fairly wide but circumscribed range of circumstances in which our society recognizes a general need to restrict the personal liberty of individual citizens either for the person's own protection or for the protection of other individuals or of society in general. Restriction of liberty is usually accompanied by the provision of special forms of care, treatment, training or occupation. . . .'

The mentally disordered were not the only social group to whom this applied. The criminal law made provisions for preventive detention or corrective training. Compulsion could be applied to persons suffering from, or suspected suffering from, infectious diseases. Sick or infirm persons could be

[1] 'A barbarous expression signifying that legally they are no longer designated under the Lunacy and Mental Treatment Acts, and are not obliged to observe the procedures laid down in the Acts.' Op. cit. para. 225.

compulsorily removed under certain circumstances laid down in section 47 of the National Assistance Act; and legislation concerned with education and child care involved compulsion in the interests of the child. The principle was thus a general one, and there was no reason why a special stigma should be thought to operate in the case of mental disorder.

The use of special compulsory powers on the grounds of mental disorder was justified on four criteria:

(1) That the patient was suffering from a recognizable and treatable form of mental disorder.

(2) That suitable care could not be provided without the use of compulsion.

(3) That the patient was unwilling to receive care without the use of compulsion.[1]

(4) *Either* that there was a good prospect of improvement in the patient's condition as a result of care and treatment.

Or that there was a strong case for using compulsory powers in order to protect others from the patient's anti-social behaviour.

The general procedures recommended for compulsion involved a streamlining of existing procedures, but without the intervention of a magistrate. Three main procedures were suggested: admission for observation, up to twenty-eight days; admission for treatment; and emergency admission. In the first two cases, the application would be made by a relative (not necessarily the nearest relative, though the nearest relative would have a special power of discharge) or a mental welfare officer of the local health authority, and would be supported by two medical recommendations, in the last case, one medical recommendation was sufficient; but the duration of an emergency order would be only seventy-two hours, and it would lapse unless the second medical certificate was added during that time'

In the same way that the concept of voluntary treatment, developed historically in connection with the mentally ill, was in future to be applied to the mentally defective also, the concept of guardianship, developed for mental defectives, was to be applicable to the mentally ill. This theme was not developed in the Report; but the general assimilation of the two previous systems of procedure into one system, to be used for both categories of patients, meant that this would become a possibility in suitable cases. Guardianship rights and duties might be vested in private individuals or in local health authorities as an alternative to in-patient treatment, and would involve the same procedures for the use of compulsion.

Special safeguards were recommended where psychopaths were concerned. This question involved a difficult issue, for, as the Report comments:

'If one concentrates on the patient's behaviour rather than on the mental

---

[1] A curious phrase is used here—'and there is at least a strong likelihood that his unwillingness is due to a lack of appreciation of his own condition deriving from the mental disorder itself'. This would seem to be difficult to state categorically.

conditions which lie behind it, one comes very close to making certain forms of behaviour in themselves grounds for segregation from society, which almost amounts to the creation of new criminal offences.'

Evidence that the person concerned was a drug addict, an alcoholic, or a sexual pervert was not in itself sufficient grounds for the use of compulsion, unless his anti-social acts offended against the criminal code. It was therefore agreed that compulsion should be limited to the duration of an observation order (twenty-eight days) in patients over the age of twenty-one. Patients who were first admitted under a treatment order before that age should be liable to compulsory detention up to the age of twenty-five, but not beyond that age. Compulsion should in any case only be used under the general criteria set out in paragraph 317—which included the proviso that there must be a good prospect of improvement in the patient's condition as a result of care and treatment. It was recognized that this would probably only apply to some psychopaths, since in the present state of psychiatric knowledge, prospects of cure or improvement varied greatly. After outlining experiments in the treatment of psychopaths at Rampton, where training for 'moral defectives' was carried out under conditions of strict security, and at Belmont, where the methods of psychotherapy and group therapy were used in a therapeutic community setting, the Report concluded:

'It is known that some psychopathic patients respond to each of these methods and some do not. It is also known that some of them . . . respond to the punitive and deterrent effect of normal penal processes in much the same way as more normal people, though others do not.'

The use of compulsion in the case of a psychopath must thus be linked not only to his age (since the prospects of success in training were greatest before his patterns of behaviour were fully formed) but also to the prognosis in his particular case in view of the resources available.

Power of discharge in the case of all patients admitted under compulsion should be held by the patient's nearest relative, subject to a barring certificate as under section 74 of the Lunacy Act 1890. A difference is that under the 1890 Act, the medical officer of the institution was to certify in a barring certificate that the patient was 'dangerous and unfit to be at large'. The new phraseology was 'dangerous to himself or to others'. Power of discharge should also be held by the medical superintendent, any three members of the Hospital Management Committee of the Board of Governors and the Mental Health Review Tribunal for the area; and a reserve power should be held by the Minister of Health. The Board of Control had recommended that this reserve power of discharge should be held at central level by a body of independent commissioners; but the Royal Commission pointed out that when the Mental Health Review Tribunals were in operation, much of the work of the central authority would be of a purely routine nature. It was therefore preferable that this should be carried out in a part-time capacity by officials who had other work to do, since full-time occupation on duties of this kind would not be such as to attract workers of high calibre.

(iv) Court Cases

There have always been points of contact between lunacy law and criminal law where persons whose mental disorder brings them into conflict with the criminal code are concerned. It was recommended that there should be an extension of the existing procedures for transferring such people to mental hospitals or mental deficiency institutions. Under section 4 of the Criminal Justice Act, 1948, patients might be required to enter mental hospital on a voluntary basis as a condition of probation; under sections 8 and 9 of the Mental Deficiency Act, 1913, and section 30 of the Magistrates' Court Act, 1930, they might be dealt with purely on the grounds of mental disorder, with no reference to the offence committed. The Commission was anxious here that mental treatment should not be regarded as a 'soft option', a way of escaping the due process of the law in doubtful cases; and that both elements—the offence and the mental condition which caused it, should be kept in mind. They therefore suggested that there should be three methods at the disposal of the Courts: they should be able to use ordinary penal measures under the criminal law, or the measures laid down by the Children and Young Persons' Acts if they considered these appropriate. They felt that there were some cases where prison, probation, or an Approved School in the case of a young person, might be the most suitable method of treatment in the interests of society and of the patient. Secondly, they should be able to direct the provision of hospital treatment or community care, with or without compulsion. Third, if they felt that there was a real danger that the patient would commit 'further and serious offences' if discharged prematurely, a Court of Quarter Sessions or Assize should be able to stipulate the period of treatment. Such a patient could then only be discharged in a shorter period with the consent of the Home Secretary. If the hospital or local authority wished to discharge him before that period was up, the patient would be referred back to the Court.

The general effect of these recommendations would be to increase the range of methods at the disposal of the Courts, and to enable them to keep both factors—mental disorder and the offence—in mind simultaneously. Existing provisions presented a clear-cut alternative in which the patient must be treated either as a fully-responsible criminal or as a totally irresponsible person suffering from mental disorder. The Commission felt that there were many grades between the two, and left the task of deciding the position in an individual case to the Courts.

Recommendations concerning 'Broadmoor' patients were outside the Commission's terms of reference; but they suggested that consideration should be given to the question of whether Broadmoor procedures could be assimilated to those for other patients. They disliked the term 'Broadmoor patient' as it referred to persons arraigned before the higher courts and found 'insane on arraignment' or 'guilty but insane', and suggested that it might well fall into disuse together with such terms as 'lunatic' and 'idiot'.

BIBLIOGRAPHY

Public General Statutes

5 and 6 Vict., c. 87	Lunatic Asylums Act, 1842.
8 and 9 Vict., c. 100	Lunatics Act, 1845.
16 and 17 Vict., c. 70	Lunacy Regulation Act, 1853.
16 and 17 Vict., c. 96	Lunatics Care and Treatment Amendment Act, 1853.
16 and 17 Vict., c. 97	Lunatic Asylums Amendment Act, 1853.
21 and 22 Vict., c. 90	Medical Registration Act, 1858.
25 and 26 Vict., c. 111	Lunatics Law Amendment Act, 1862.
49 and 50 Vict., c. 25	Idiots Act, 1886.
52 and 53 Vict., c. 41	Lunatics Law Amendment Act, 1889.
53 Vict., c. 5	Lunacy (Consolidation) Act 1890.
54 and 55 Vict., c. 65	Lunacy Act, 1891.
62 and 63 Vict., c. 32	Elementary Education (Defective and Epileptic Children) Act, 1899.
3 and 4 Geo. V, c. 28	Mental Deficiency Act, 1913.
4 and 5 Geo. V, c. 45	Elementary Education (Defective and Epileptic Children) Act, 1914.
17 and 18 Geo. V, c. 33	Mental Deficiency Act, 1927.
19 Geo. V, c. 17	Local Government Act, 1929.
20 and 21 Geo. V, c. 23	Mental Treatment Act, 1930.
9 and 10 Geo. VI, c. 81	National Health Service Act, 1946.
7 and 8 Eliz. II, c. 72	Mental Health Act, 1959.

Unpassed Bills

Lunacy Acts Amendment Bill, 1887.
Lunacy Bill, 1887.
Feeble-Minded Control Bill, 1912.
Mental Defect Bill, 1912.
Mental Treatment Bill, 1915.

Official Papers (Published by H. M. Stationery Office)

Hansard's Parliamentary Debates.
House of Commons Journal, 1845–96.
Reports of Select Committees of the House of Commons:
  On Lunatics, 1859–60.
  On the Operation of Lunacy Law, 1877–8.

Reports of Royal Commissions:

  On the Care of the Feeble-Minded, 1908 (the Radnor Commission).

BIBLIOGRAPHY

On the Poor Laws, 1909.
On Lunacy and Mental Disorder, 1926 (the MacMillan Commission).
On the Laws Relating to Mental Illness and Mental Deficiency, 1957.

Reports of Official Committees:

Ministry of Health—Departmental Committee on the Administration of Public Mental Hospitals, 1922.
Board of Education and Board of Control: Joint Committee on Mental Deficiency, 1929 (Wood Report).
Ministry of Health—Departmental Committee on Sterilization, 1934 (Brock Report).
Ministry of Health—Departmental Committee on the Voluntary Mental Health Services, 1939 (Feversham Report).
Inter-departmental Committee on Social Insurance and Allied Services, 1942 (Beveridge Report).
Annual Reports of the Lunacy Commissioners, 1845–1912.
Annual Reports of the Board of Control, 1913–58.
Annual Reports of the Ministry of Health, 1949–58.
Ministry of Health and Board of Control: The National Health Service Act, 1946: Provisions Relating to the Mental Health Services, 1948.
Central Health Services Council: Report on Co-operation between Hospital, Local Authority and General Practitioner Services, 1952.
Board of Control: Report of Conference on the Mental Treatment Act, 1930.
Colonies for Mental Defectives, 1931.
A Study of Hypoglycaemic Shock Treatment in Schizophrenia, 1936.
Suggestions and Instructions for the Arrangement . . . of Mental Hospitals, 1940.
Pre-frontal Leucotomy in 1,000 cases, 1947.

Journals

Biometrika.
British Medical Journal.
Hansard's Parliamentary Debates.
International Journal of Social Psychiatry.
Journal of Mental Science, formerly *Asylum Journal, Asylum Journal of Mental Science.*
Journal of Psychological Medicine.
Lancet.
Mental Health.

Unpublished Papers (in manuscript)

Minutes of the Council of the Eugenics Education Society, 1907–12.
Minutes of the Manchester Branch of the Eugenics Education Society, 1912.
Private Papers of Dame Ellen Pinsent (by kind permission of Lady Adrian).
Private Papers of the Eugenics Society and the National Association for the Care of the Feeble-Minded. (By kind permission of the Eugenics Society.)
A. J. Willcocks, Interest-Groups and the National Health Service Act, 1946. (Ph.D. thesis in the Library of the University of Birmingham, presented October, 1953.)

Books, Pamphlets and Articles

ALLEGED LUNATICS' FRIEND SOCIETY. *Annual Reports.*
ASHDOWN, M. and BROWN, S. C. *Social Service and Mental Health* (Routledge and Kegan Paul, London, 1953).
ASSOCIATION FOR PSYCHIATRIC SOCIAL WORKERS. *Training for Social Work.* n.d.
Asylum for Idiots, Park House, Highgate. Brochure published London, 1847.

BIBLIOGRAPHY

ATLAY, J. B. *The Victorian Chancellors* (Smith, Elder, London, 1906–8).

BARR, A. W. *Mental Defectives: Their History, Treatment and Training* (Rebman, London, 1904).

Bethlem Hospital. Brochure prepared for the official opening of the new buildings, July 1930.

BICKMORE, A. *Industries for the Feeble-Minded* (Bartholomew Press, London, 1913).

BIERER, J. *The Day Hospital* (H. K. Lewis, London, 1951).

—*Therapeutic Social Clubs* (H. K. Lewis, London n.d.).

BOSANQUET, H. *Social Work in London—A History of the Charity Organization Society* (Murray, London, 1914).

CARSE, J. *The Worthing Experiment* (South-west Metropolitan Regional Hospital Board, 1958).

CATTELL, J. MCKEEN. 'Address before the American Psychological Association', *Psychological Review*, vol. III, 2.

CENTRAL ASSOCIATION FOR THE CARE OF THE MENTALLY DEFECTIVE. *Annual Reports, 1915–23.*

CENTRAL ASSOCIATION FOR MENTAL WELFARE. *Annual Reports, 1924–44.*

CHARITY ORGANIZATION SOCIETY. *Report of Sub-Committee on The Education and Care of Idiots, Imbeciles and Harmless Lunatics* (Charity Organization Series, 1877).

CLOUSTON, T. 'Training Course in Psychiatry', *J. Ment. Sci.* (April, 1911).

COLLINS, W. *The Woman in White*, 1st ed. 1869 (Collins Classics, 1952).

CONOLLY, J. *An Inquiry Concerning the Indications of Insanity* (London, 1830).

—*On the Treatment of Insanity* (London, 1856).

COOPER, BERYL P. *Minds Matter: A New Approach to Mental Health* (Bow Group, Conservative Political Centre, 1958).

CURRAN, D. and GUTTMAN, E. *Psychological Medicine*, 3rd ed. 1949 (Livingstone, Edinburgh).

DENDY, M. see Lapage, C. P.

DREIKAUS, R. 'Group Psychotherapy and the Third Revolution in Psychiatry', *Int. Journal Soc. Psychiatry*, vol. I, 3.

DREIKAUS, R. and CORSINI. 'Twenty Years of Group Psychotherapy', *Am. J. Psych.* (Feb. 1954).

DUGDALE, R.L. *The Jukes: A Study in Crime, Disease and Heredity, 1877.* 4th ed. 1910 (Putnam, London and New York)

ELLIS, SIR WILLIAM C. *A Treatise on the Nature, Causes, Symptoms and Treatment of Insanity* (London, 1838).

ESTABROOK, A. H. *The Jukes in 1915* (Carnegie Institute of Washington, 1916).

EUGENICS EDUCATION SOCIETY, *Annual Reports*, 1908–26.

EUGENICS SOCIETY, *Annual Reports*, 1926–54.

FLÜGEL, J. C. *A Hundred Years of Psychology* (Duckworth, London, 1933).

FOULKES, S. H. and ANTHONY, E. J. *Group Psychotherapy: the Psychoanalytic Approach* (Pelican Books, London, 1957).

GALTON, SIR FRANCIS. *Hereditary Genius* (London, 1869).

—'Local Associations for Promoting Eugenics', *Nature*, Oct. 22nd, 1908.

—*Natural Inheritance* (London, 1889).

—*The Problem of the Feeble-Minded* (London, 1909).

GODDARD, H. *The Kallikak Family.* 1912

GODDARD, H. A., et al. *The Work of the Mental Nurse*, Manchester Mental Nursing Survey (Manchester University Press, 1955).

BIBLIOGRAPHY

GRENVILLE, J. MORTIMER. *The Care and Cure of the Insane*. Report of Lancet Commission London 1877.

GRICE, J. WATSON. *National and Local Finance* (London, 1910).

HAMMOND, J. L. and BARBARA. *Lord Shaftesbury*, 1923 (Pelican Books, 1939).

HARGREAVES, G. R. *Psychiatry and the Public Health*, Heath Clark Lectures, University of London (O.U.P., 1958).

HILL, R. GARDINER. *The Non-Restraint System of Treatment in Lunacy*. Simpkin Marshall, London. 1857.

HODDER, E. *Life and Work of the Seventh Earl of Shaftesbury*. 3 vols. London 1886.

HOYLE, J. S. and HAWKSWORTH, T. S. *The Mental Health Officers' Guide*. Elsworth Bros., London. 1956 Edition.

Institute of Public Administration. *The Health Services: some of their Practical Problems* (Allen and Unwin, 1951).

ITARD. *L'Education de Sauvage d'Aveyron*. 1901.

JONES, K. *Lunacy, Law and Conscience, 1744–1845* (Routledge and Kegan Paul, 1954).

—'Problems of Mental After Care in Lancashire', *Sociological Review*, July 1954.

JONES, M. *Social Psychiatry*. (Routledge and Kegan Paul, 1952).

JOHNSON, K. J. 'Bethlem and the Maudsley', *Bethlem and Maudsley Gazette*, May 1953.

KEIR, S. *The Royal Albert Institution, Lancaster*. Printed at the Institution, 1937.

KIRKBRIDE, T. *On the Construction of Hospitals for the Insane*, 2nd edition (Philadelphia, 1880).

LAPAGE, C. P. *Feeble-Mindedness in Children of School Age*, with an Appendix on Sandlebridge by Mary Dendy (Manchester University Press, 1920).

LEADBITTER, A. *Heredity and the Social Problem Group* (Arnold, 1933).

LOMAX, M. *Experiences of an Asylum Doctor*, 1921.

MAYER-GROSS, W., SLATER, E., and ROTH, M. *Clinical Psychiatry* (Cassell, 1954).

MCKENNA, S. *Reginald McKenna, 1863–1943* (Eyre and Spottiswoode, 1948).

MEAD, M. (ed.) *Cultural Patterns and Technical Change*. U.N.E.S.C.O. 1955.

Medical Officer: 'Change in Mental Hospital—A Therapeutic Community', articles in the *Manchester Guardian*, January 28th and 29th, 1959.

Mental After-Care Association. *Annual Report*, 1951.

Two explanatory pamphlets untitled, n.d.

MORRIS, C. (ed.) *Social Case-Work in Great Britain* (Faber, 1950).

National Association for Mental Health. Reports of Annual Conferences.

Directory of Adult Out-Patient Facilities in England and Wales, 1957.

National Council for Civil Liberties. *50,000 Outside the Law*. London, n.d.

PATERNOSTER, R. *The Madhouse System* (published by the author, London, 1841).

PEARSON, KARL. *The Life, Letters and Labours of Francis Galton*, 4 vols. (Cambridge University Press, 1914).

PENROSE, L.S. *The Biology of Mental Defect* (Sidgwick and Jackson, 1949).

PINSENT, DAME ELLEN (Mrs. Hume Pinsent). 'On the Permanent Care of the Feeble-Minded', *Lancet*, 21st Feb. 1903.

—*The Oxford Mental Health Services* (Oxford University Press, 1937).

ROBINSON, K. *Policy for Mental Health*, Fabian Research Series pamphlet, 1958.

ROOFF, M. *Voluntary Societies and Social Policy* (Routledge and Kegan Paul, 1957).

BIBLIOGRAPHY

ROSS, J. STIRLING. *The National Health Service in Great Britain* (Oxford University Press, 1952).

Royal Medico-Psychological Association: Report of Medical Planning Committee—*A Memorandum on the Future Organisation of the Psychiatric Services* (privately printed, London 1945).

Runwell Hospital. Brochure prepared for the official opening of the hospital, 1937.

SELBOURNE. Roundell Palmer, 1st Earl of Selborne. *Memoirs Personal and Political, 1865–1895* (Macmillan, London, 1898).

STIRLING ROSS, see Ross, J. Stirling.

Surrey Asylum. *Rules of Surrey Asylum*, printed together with Reports of the Visiting Justices, 1844–6 (London, 1847).

TITMUSS, R. *Problems of Social Policy*. History of World War II. U.K. Civil Series, H.M.S.O and Longmans, 1950.

TREDGOLD, A. F. *Mental Deficiency*, 1st ed. 1908, 7th ed. 1947 (Ballière Tindall and Cox).

TUKE, D. H. *Chapters in the History of the Insane in the British Isles* (Kegan Paul, 1882).

WATSON GRICE, see Grice.

WEBB, S. *Grants in Aid* (London, 1911).

WEDGWOOD, J. *Memoirs of a Fighting Life*, 1940.

WELFARE, MARJORIE U. *Dame Evelyn Fox*. Pamphlet reprinted from *Social Service*, Spring. 1955.

WORMALD, J. and WORMALD, S. *A Guide to the Mental Deficiency Act*, 1913 (King, London, 1913).

INDEX

INDEX

INDEX

Institute of Psychiatry, 104
Intelligence-testing, 49–51
Itard, Dr., 43–4

Jackson, Mr. R. M., 183
James, (Sir) Archibald, 90 and n.
Jane Eyre, 20–21, 22
Joint Health Consultative Committees, 156–7
Jones, Dr. Maxwell, 168
Journal of Mental Science, 12
Jowitt, Lord, 107, 118
Juke Family, 51–2, 59
Justice's Order, *see* Magistrate's Order

Kallikak Family, 51–2, 59
Kekewich, S. T., 13 n.
Kilmuir, Lord, 192

Lancaster Asylum, 94
Lancet Commission, 1877, 23–5, 94
Lay Administrators, *see* Institute of Hospital Administrators
Lewis, (Prof. Sir) Aubrey, 145
Liberty of the Subject, *see* Certification, Magistrate's Order
Licenced Houses, *see* Private Asylums
Lincoln Asylum, 9, 94
Littlemore County Mental Hospital, 136–7
Local Authority Care (since 1948—*see* Mental Health Departments)
Local Government Act, 1929, 86, 115, 120 n.
Local Government Board, 99
Loch, Sir Charles, 56
Lomax, Dr. Montague, 100–1
Lucas-Tooth, Sir Hugh, M.P., 188
Lunacy Act, 1889, 17 n., 33–4
Lunacy Act, 1890, Bill in Parliament, 34: Duties of Relieving Officer under, 160: Duration of, 178: Effects of, 94, 141: Legal influence on, 10, 40, 93, 192: and magistrate's order, 17 n.: and mental defectives, 43: and Mental Deficiency Act, 1913, 72: Terms, 35–40, 97, 120, 221

Lunacy Acts Amendment Bill, 1887, 32
Lunacy Acts Amendment Bill, 1888–9, 32–4
Lunacy Amendment Bill, 1885, 31
Lunacy Bill, 1883, 30
Lunacy Bill, 1887, 32
Lunacy Commissioners, 8, 14, 16–9, 25, 35–40, 46, 69, 207: *see also* Board of Control
Lunacy Laws Amendment Association, 26, 29
Lunatics Act, 1845, 1–3, 7–11, 19, 38

Macadam, Miss Elizabeth, 129
Mackinnon, Lord, 107
Mackintosh Committee, Report, 143, 159–60, 163
McKenna, Rt. Hon. Reginald, Home Secretary, 63, 64, 65
Maclay, Dr. the Hon. W. S., 211, 212
Macmillan, Lord, 107, 118: Report, *see* Royal Commission, 1924–6
Madhouse Act, 1828, 7 n., 8, 18, 37
Magistrate's Order in Certification of Mentally Ill, 8, 17, 23, 25, 32–3, 35–7, 186, 197, 213: *see also* Certification
Manchester Lunatic Hospital, *see* Cheadle Royal
Married Women's Property Act, 27
Maudsley Hospital, 93, 103–4, 104 n., 145, 151
Maudsley, Sir Henry, 103–4
Mechanical Restraint, 38
Medical Officer of Mental Health, 86, 139
Medical Planning Commission, 1940, 147
Medical Registration Act, 1858, 10, 15
Medical Research Council, *see* Research
Medical Superintendents, 94, 146, 169–71 and n.
Medico-Psychological Association, *see* Royal Medico-Psychological Association
Mellish, Mr. R. J., M.P., 181

232

For Product Safety Concerns and Information please contact our EU
representative GPSR@taylorandfrancis.com
Taylor & Francis Verlag GmbH, Kaufingerstraße 24, 80331 München, Germany